HATHA YOGA
illustrated

Martin Kirk • Brooke Boon • Daniel Di Turo

photographs by Daniel DiTuro

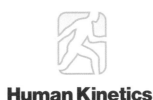

Human Kinetics

Library of Congress Cataloging-in-Publication Data

Kirk, Martin.
  Hatha yoga illustrated / Martin Kirk, Brooke Boon ; photography by
Daniel DiTuro.
      p. cm.
Includes bibliographical references.
  ISBN 0-7360-6203-3 (soft cover)
  1. Yoga, Hatha. I. Boon, Brooke. II. Title.
  RA781.7.K548 2006
  613.7'046--dc22

                                                            2005011231

ISBN-10: 0-7360-6203-3

ISBN-13: 978-0-7360-6203-9

Copyright © 2006, 2004 by Martin Kirk, Brooke Boon, and Daniel DiTuro

The Web addresses cited in this text were current as of July 14, 2005, unless otherwise noted.

Our thanks to Ted Czukor for providing the text and information on mudras in chapter 1 and many of the resources on pages 218-219.

Acquisitions Editor: Martin Barnard; **Developmental Editor:** Julie Rhoda; **Assistant Editors:** Carla Zych, Alisha Jeddeloh, Wendy McLaughlin; **Copyeditor:** Lisa Morgan; **Proofreader:** Pam Johnson; **Graphic Designer:** Robert Reuther; **Graphic Artist:** Tara Welsch; **Photo Manager:** Dan Wendt; **Cover Designer:** Keith Blomberg; **Photographer (cover and interior):** Daniel DiTuro; **Art Manager:** Kareema McLendon; **Illustrator:** concept by Nora and Ted Czukor, redrawn by Kareema McLendon-Foster

Human Kinetics books are available at special discounts for bulk purchase. Special editions or book excerpts can also be created to specification. For details, contact the Special Sales Manager at Human Kinetics.

Printed in Hong Kong   10   9   8

Human Kinetics
Web site: www.HumanKinetics.com

United States: Human Kinetics
P.O. Box 5076
Champaign, IL 61825-5076
800-747-4457
e-mail: humank@hkusa.com

Canada: Human Kinetics
475 Devonshire Road, Unit 100
Windsor, ON N8Y 2L5
800-465-7301 (in Canada only)
e-mail: info@hkcanada.com

Europe: Human Kinetics
107 Bradford Road
Stanningley
Leeds LS28 6AT, United Kingdom
+44 (0)113 255 5665
e-mail: hk@hkeurope.com

Australia: Human Kinetics
57A Price Avenue
Lower Mitcham, South Australia 5062
08 8372 0999
e-mail: info@hkaustralia.com

New Zealand: Human Kinetics
Division of Sports Distributors NZ Ltd.
P.O. Box 300 226 Albany
North Shore City, Auckland
0064 9 448 1207
e-mail: info@humankinetics.co.nz

HATHA YOGA
illustrated

To my wife, Jordan Kirk, with whom I share the journey of teaching yoga, and to my teachers John Friend and Douglas Brooks

Martin Kirk

For my husband, Jarrett, and my beautiful children, Jory, Jace, and Brynn

Brooke Boon

To Brenda and Brandy

Daniel DiTuro

Contents

Preface

A journey of a thousand miles begins with a single step.

Chinese proverb

Similarly, the journey to write and illustrate this book began with a single photograph shot in February 1999. Like many events in life, it was unplanned. I had been practicing hatha yoga for about six months and was already sold on its therapeutic benefits. When the model I was photographing sat cross-legged on the floor and arranged her flowing dress around her, I asked her to place her hands in Namaste (prayer position) and close her eyes. I titled the photograph Namaste. It is still one of my favorite photographs from what would eventually evolve into The Yoga Project, a photographic work with a mission to inspire and enlighten people about the mental, physical, and spiritual benefits of yoga.

As my journey of yoga continued, I was surprised and disturbed by the many misconceptions people had about this ancient East Indian philosophy. Many of my friends mistakenly believed it was a religion and insisted they would never practice yoga because it would interfere with their religious beliefs. Many male friends insisted that guys don't do yoga. I shared my yoga photographs with them, illustrating the true nature of the yoga practice, emphasizing that yoga is not aligned with a specific religious practice but that it is inclusive of all people. Some were amazed, others were intrigued, and yet others remained skeptical. It became clear to me then that much more needed to be done to educate people about the real mental and physical benefits of yoga—especially hatha yoga, the practice of physical yoga postures. Although hatha yoga is a small branch of all the yoga practices, it has become the Yoga Project's main emphasis due to its popularity in the West. Additionally, the Yoga Project works to inform and educate people about meditation and pranayama.

Hatha yoga can calm the mind, provide a gentle workout, or make you sweat. It can reduce your heart rate when you are stressed or elevate it by providing a vigorous workout. Many refer to it as a New Age practice, yet its origin dates back thousands of years.

Whether you are new to the practice of hatha yoga, or simply curious about it, this book provides practical, detailed information you can use throughout your daily life and in your yoga practice. Chapter 1 provides background information about yoga and how to get the most out of your yoga practice. Chapters 2 through 10 then provide detailed information for 77 asanas classified by the type of posture. Included are standing postures, balancing postures, arm-balance postures, inverted postures, backward-bending postures, twisting postures, forward-bending postures, sitting postures, and reclining and relaxation postures. Each asana has photographs depicting the starting, intermediate, and final positions accompanied by detailed step-by-step instructions. In addition, you will learn about the asanas' mental and physical benefits, contraindications, counterposes, and gazing points (drishtis). Most asanas include a gentle variation for beginning, less flexible, or physically challenged students as well as variation postures to enhance your yoga practice. Chapter 11 illustrates 11 hatha yoga routines ranging from a very gentle routine, consisting primarily of supported postures, to more vigorous vinyasa (flow) yoga, including the Sun and Moon Salutations, in which you proceed from one posture to the next with little or no rest.

There are many schools of hatha yoga. Each school offers something unique. Unlike many other forms of physical activity and spiritual practice there is a level and style of hatha yoga for almost everyone. Authors Martin Kirk and Brooke Boon are both certified instructors in the Anusara and Baptiste Power Yoga schools, respectively.

Sanskrit, the ancient Indian language in which the original yoga texts were written, is used throughout this book. If you are new to yoga, do not be intimidated by the Sanskrit words. As your journey to yoga progresses, learning some of the Sanskrit terms and posture names will enhance the journey and not impede it. If the only Sanskrit words you ever learn are asana (posture) and Namaste (the light in me honors the light in you) you will have taken one of the steps on your yoga journey.

Namaste,
Daniel DiTuro

Acknowledgments

I would like to thank God for the gift of yoga. I have been blessed with a passion for teaching and am so grateful for the ability to share that passion through works such as these. I am always amazed at how we are used in our lives if we surrender what we think we should be to the Creator and Perfector of all things. Only then are we free to become exactly what we were created to be; big, bright, purposeful, relevant beings. I am appreciative of the abundance that I have received through trust and faith.

A special thank you to my coauthors Martin and Jordan for their expertise, willingness to combine efforts, and unwavering dedication, and to Daniel for his photographic talent.

To my husband, Jarrett, and my children, Jory, Jace, and Brynn, the greatest joys in my life. Thank you for seeing me through deadlines and sleepless nights when I was less than agreeable. I appreciate your unconditional love and respect for my personal growth and for seeing in me all that I am now only beginning to see in myself. Mostly, thank you God for giving my life meaning and using me for Your glory.

Brooke Boon

To my beloved wife and partner in teaching, Jordan, who came into my life and gave me the courage to take the bold step from engineering designer of space satellite electronics to full time yogi. She is the one who deserves the credit for this work with her tireless writing, critiquing, and editing the asana descriptions and spotting and directing the photo sessions. This book would not have been possible without her. She is ever my beloved teacher and friend.

To my teacher, John Friend, for the gift of Anusara Yoga. John gives so freely of himself to others and inspires us all to do the same: He is truly the friend of the universe.

To my philosophy teacher and mentor, Professor Douglas Brooks, who helped with scholarly details for the book and who has provided guidance and amazing wisdom from the day we first met.

To my coauthor, Brooke, for graciously accommodating the differences in our styles and wholeheartedly embracing our work together as a team.

Thanks to Daniel DiTuro for the excellent photographic and coordination work that allowed Brooke and me to write this book.

Mostly, I want to thank my mother and father for always being willing to answer my questions and expose me to new ideas. They have always encouraged me to follow my heart.

Martin Kirk

This book would not have been possible without the support of dozens of people who dedicated hundreds of hours to bring an idea to reality. First, I must thank Brenda Godfrey, friend, model, makeup artist, hair stylist, and photographer, who inspired the creation of the Yoga Project which eventually lead to writing and photographing this book. A book of this magnitude is not possible without models. Brandy Maktima was one of the original Yoga Project models and a principal model for this book. A special thank you to Brandy's husband, Tony, who cared for their children while Mom was modeling. Pamela Scott modeled the alternate nostril breathing sequence.

An instructional book about hatha yoga required the knowledge of highly trained and certified yoga instructors. My coauthors, Martin and Brooke, contributed their expertise and insight for the benefit of current and future yogis. This book would not have been possible without them.

Wayne Johnson and Debbie Forrestt have both greatly contributed to my knowledge of yoga. Wayne, I am glad you decided to teach yoga and for your advice, critique, and assistance photographing the supported postures in this book. Om Shantih, Wayne. Thank you, Debbie, for convincing me that 98 percent accuracy was not good enough. Many people worked behind the scenes to create the photographs for this book. I am grateful to Marylove Jacobs and Ann James for assisting during the photo shoots and to Jim Adair for convincing me that digital photography rules. Jordan Kirk spotted many of the active postures and modeled vinyasa yoga routines II and III. Her knowledge, time, and efforts modeling, selecting many of the photos appearing in the book, and editing the manuscript are greatly appreciated. My thanks to the staff at Hugger Mugger Yoga Products for their assistance in selecting many of the props used to photograph the asanas in this book.

A very special thank you to Martin Barnard, Julie Rhoda, and Dan Wendt of Human Kinetics for their support, guidance, and assistance in bringing a concept to reality.

Daniel DiTuro

Introduction

Welcome to the practice of yoga. With this book you begin a wonderful journey of discovery into your body and yourself that will help you find your fullest potential physically, mentally, emotionally, and spiritually. Whether you come to yoga in search of greater strength and flexibility, physical healing, or a deeper understanding of life, this great path has something to offer you. For thousands of years, travelers have trod this inward path before you, so the trail is well marked. Your own yoga journey will be as individual as you are, but you will never travel alone. You will become part of a great caravan of grace among others who seek to enrich their lives and make the world a better place.

Anyone can benefit from the practice of yoga. People of all ages, backgrounds, cultures, and religions come to yoga. Some are in great health; others come with injuries or physical limitations. Some travel for a brief distance along the path; others embrace the journey as a lifelong pursuit. This great practice is big enough for everyone with the desire to improve their health and learn to live life from a place of joy and adventure. Regardless of your starting point, there is no doubt that you will meet many like-minded travelers on your journey. Yoga is enjoying an unprecedented surge in popularity in the West, with an estimated sixteen million Americans practicing some form of yoga. There are classes for all levels and a variety of different styles from which to choose. You can begin your journey from right where you are today in the manner that speaks most to your heart.

This book serves as an introduction to yoga for many and as a guidebook to continue the journey for others. The majority of the information provided concerns the physical postures of yoga, the *asanas*. Each asana contains detailed information about getting into the pose, finding proper alignment, and obtaining the greatest benefit from your practice. Introductions are also provided into the practices of *pranayama* (yogic breathing), *mudras* (yoga of the hands), and meditation. Any of these practices can be helpful to you in your life. Taken together, these great practices can be quite transformational.

Most Westerners think of yoga as the set of postures and breathing exercises known as *hatha* or "sun and moon" yoga. This is the physical yoga practice that uses body postures to open the body and heart. But yoga is much more than a physical practice. The science of yoga is thousands of years old. It is an entire system with its own set of moral codes, breathing disciplines, and meditation techniques designed to take you along your spiritual journey.

The word *yoga* is classically translated as "union." It is a drawing together of heart, mind, and body that integrates all the parts of ourselves into a unified whole. Just as a team performs at its best when all the members line up behind a common goal, we will be at our best when every part of ourselves is in alignment with every other part. We are happiest when we are following our hearts and doing what we really love. In essence, when we bring our hearts, minds, and bodies into alignment, we step into the flow of grace that is yoga. The journey of yoga is an inward search to find the very best within us and then to learn to express that every day in our bodies, minds, and hearts.

Many of the practices we see in modern yoga are quite old, while others are surprisingly young. The physical yoga we know today as *hatha* is not even mentioned in the earliest yoga texts. Yoga has always evolved to meet the needs of the people and the time. In fact, many of today's hatha yoga postures are less than one hundred years old. They can be traced to Tirumalai Krishnamacharya, a five-foot, two-inch South Indian man born in 1888 in a small Indian village. Krishnamacharya learned yoga from his father as a young man and decided to teach it to others. *Hatha* yoga was not well known in India in those days, however, and his early teaching years were a struggle for financial survival. Then in the 1930s he was given the position of teaching yoga at the gymnastics hall of the royal palace. His students were primarily active young boys bustling with energy, and Krishnamacharya knew he had to keep them busy. So he borrowed from the disciplines of gymnastics and Indian wrestling to produce a dynamic series of postures that would fit their active demeanor. His series of asanas still persists today and is known as *Ashtanga Vinyasa Yoga*, a system popularized by one of his primary students, Pattabai Jois. Yoga continues to evolve. The skillful use of alignment in the yoga asanas was mastered and shared with the world by B.K.S. Iyengar, another well-known and highly respected student of Krishnamacharya, who, in his eighties, still teaches yoga today. And many former students of B.K.S. Iyengar, now well-known instructors in their own right, continue to innovate to this day (John Friend, Rodney Yee, Angela Farmer, Victor Van Hooten, and others).

The asana descriptions in this book are primarily based on a set of alignment principles developed by John Friend, founder of Anusara Yoga. These principles have helped thousands—beginners and seasoned students alike—to take their practices to new levels while supporting sound alignment of body, mind, and heart. Additionally, they have been used with great success for the treatment and prevention of injuries.

The documented medical benefits of yoga include increased strength and stamina, relief of stress and anxiety, and lowered blood pressure. Most students find that they feel better with a regular practice of yoga in their lives. Whether you are seeking to improve your athletic performance, heal an old injury, or increase your flexibility, you will find the practice of yoga to be filled with rich traditions and meaning that can enhance your quality of life. And do not measure your success in yoga by how well you are able to do a particular pose. Just enjoy the ride. For with yoga, as with any worthwhile undertaking, the joy is in the journey, not the destination.

Enjoy your yoga journey.

chapter 1

Art and Practice of Hatha Yoga

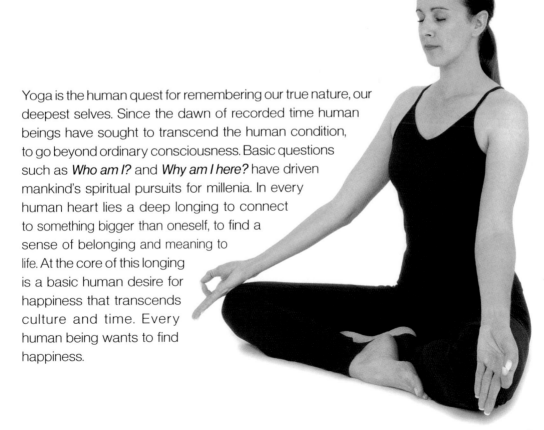

Yoga is the human quest for remembering our true nature, our deepest selves. Since the dawn of recorded time human beings have sought to transcend the human condition, to go beyond ordinary consciousness. Basic questions such as *Who am I?* and *Why am I here?* have driven mankind's spiritual pursuits for millenia. In every human heart lies a deep longing to connect to something bigger than oneself, to find a sense of belonging and meaning to life. At the core of this longing is a basic human desire for happiness that transcends culture and time. Every human being wants to find happiness.

This quest for happiness is not so much a striving to acquire something that exists outside of us as it is an innate desire to *remember* something that is part of our very nature. First and foremost, yoga is about remembering ourselves, our own deepest purpose for being. The journey of yoga is an inner journey to the very essence of our existence. The message of yoga is that the nature of that inner essence is happiness or bliss (*ananda* in Sanskrit). The search for happiness within every human heart is the search for the true nature of who we are.

Nowhere on earth has the impulse to transcend the human condition been more consistent and creative than in India—home to an overwhelming variety of spiritual beliefs, practices, and approaches designed to help the spiritual seeker achieve higher levels of consciousness. The practice of yoga is deeply woven into the rich Indian culture and evolved from the same roots as many other spiritual practices. As an ancient science, it was designed to facilitate the seeker's inner journey to a higher level of being.

Though the art of yoga is often associated with Hinduism, yoga is not a religion. While a religion emphasizes belief structures about life and the human relationship to the divine, yoga seeks to reveal our own deepest nature through direct experience of our divinity. One need not be religious to practice yoga, nor does yoga exclude any religious practice. All that is required to practice yoga is a desire to learn more about yourself and your relationship to the universe.

The Sanskrit word *yoga* means "union" or "yoking" and has been defined as the union of mind and body, heart and actions. The type of yoga that most Westerners recognize is the series of physical postures, or *asanas,* that strengthens and makes the body more flexible. This form of yoga is referred to as *hatha* yoga. But hatha yoga is much more than just a physical practice. The word *hatha* is a Sanskrit combination of the word *ha* (sun) and *tha* (moon), which is itself a union of opposites. Qualities associated with the sun are heat, masculinity, and effort, while moon qualities are coolness, femininity, and surrender. Hatha yoga is designed to help us bring pairs of opposites together in our hearts, minds, and bodies for the purpose of discovering something deeper about the nature of our existence. John Friend, founder of Anusara Yoga, refers to these opposites as stepping stones on a path of grace. They are qualities of heart such as effort and surrender, courage and contentment, stillness and playfulness. They may also be physical qualities such as hard and soft, hot and cold, solid and flowing. In essence, the practice of yoga brings together apparent opposites into a harmonious union—a place in the middle.

This middle place is a gateway into a whole new world for most of us. It is a place where we discover wonderful new things about our abilities and possibilities for our lives. It is a gateway into our own hearts. When we step through this gateway we do not step alone. We find before us the footprints of many who have gone before and illuminated the path. We find ourselves in the current of a great river that has carried the hopes and dreams of many seekers over the centuries. There is power in the river that will help us along our own spiritual journey, the power of grace. And by stepping through that gateway into the currents of grace, the yogi steps forward into ever-greater possibilities of his or her own happiness and self-expression.

Roots of Yoga

The earliest recorded form of yoga was a deeply introspective and meditative practice that focused on sacrificial rituals. Yoga is first mentioned in the *Vedas*, a body of four sacred texts that are the oldest and most treasured scriptures of the sacred canon of Hinduism. It is in the oldest of these scriptures, the *Ṛg* (pronounced rig) *Veda*, where the word yoga and its root, *yuj*, which means "yoke," first appear. However, at that time no systematic path of yoga yet existed.

Most scholars believe the *Vedas* were composed by Sanskrit-speaking people who arrived in the Indus Valley of what is now India somewhere between 1800 and 1500 B.C.E. It is not clear whether these people, calling themselves Arya, invaded or peacefully assimilated the prevailing culture into their own, but they brought with them the earliest roots of what we now enjoy as the practice of yoga.

Veda means "knowledge" or "wisdom," and the original four texts are regarded as sacred revelations to the ancient seers (called *rishis*). They consist of literally thousands of verses of hymns and sacrificial chants designed to bring order and good fortune to those who invoke them. Two more texts, the *Brahmanas* (1000 to 800 B.C.E.) and the *Aranyakas* (800 B.C.E.), followed.

The *Vedas* and their commentaries were essentially how-to guides for ritual and sacrifice. They gave people instructions on how to make their lives better and attain success in marriage, business, war, and so forth. If you wanted to ensure success during Vedic time you would hire a priest to perform a ceremony from one of the Vedic texts.

At the end of the Vedic period (about 600 to 550 B.C.E.) there was an evolutionary leap in yogic thought with the appearance of the *Upanishads*. The *Upanishads* went beyond the instruction manual approach of the *Vedas* to ask the deeper questions about the meaning of a spiritual life.

The word *upanishad* comes from the prefixes *upa,* (approach), and *ni,* (near), and the verbal root *shad,* "to sit." It literally means "to sit nearby." The *Upanishads* serve as an invitation to come and sit near a teacher who can impart the wisdom of deeper understanding to the student. It was customary in Vedic times for students to gather around at the feet of their teacher and learn his wisdom by heart. But the *Upanishads* raised the bar for the inquiry into the mysteries of life beyond that of the Vedas. In the words of Douglas Brooks, Tantric scholar and professor of religion at the University of Rochester, the *Upanishads* were for those who wanted to "stay after school," to go deeper and ask not only how the universe works but why does it work the way it does, what is its essential nature, and what is my place in it?

For fear of whom fire burns, for fear of whom the sun shines, for fear of whom the winds, clouds and death perform their offices?

Tattrirya Upanishad

It is the deeper inquiry of the *Upanishads* that defines the evolutionary path to the yoga that we know today. Over the centuries the *Upanishads* became the sustaining original wisdom of all great yoga traditions.

The early centuries before the Christian era were rich in the development of Indian thought. Near the time when the *Upanishads* were being composed (or slightly later) the legendary sage and scholar Patanjali was compiling his list of *Yoga Sutras*. The word *sutra* is composed of two parts, *su*, meaning thread and *tra*, meaning to transcend. The *Sutras* are like pearls on a thread that helps the student to transcend. They are the threads that weave together the teacher, the teaching, and the student. The *Sutras* were composed as a list of aphorisms boiling down the yogic wisdom of the age into concise sentences that could easily be committed to memory. Their terse nature left them open to interpretation, leading to a long period of commentary and analysis that continues to this day. Patanjali's *Yoga Sutras* became the cornerstone in the system known today as Classical yoga, which is explored in greater detail in the next section.

Three Yogic World Views

In the West, yoga is often confused with Hinduism. It is understandable that people group the two together because they share a common culture, language, and terminology. Both traditions trace their roots back to the *Rg Veda*. The common basis for both traditions is the Sanskrit language. In India many Hindus practice yoga, but not all yogis are Hindu.

Yoga is a philosophical system that prescribes a way of life and is actually just one of the philosophical schools recognized by Hindu orthodoxy as a valid representation of Vedic truth. There are many such schools that have played a role in the evolution of Indian thought. Each school is a form of philosophical thought that has evolved in India throughout the centuries. Several of these systems have been exported to the West, and particularly the United States, over the years. With the recent, unprecedented rise in the popularity of hatha yoga it is important to identify the foundations on which modern yoga systems are based.

Among the exports of Indian thought, three philosophical traditions now form an essential core within contemporary yoga: Classical yoga, Advaita Vedanta, and Tantra. Every popular system of hatha yoga in the West today is grounded in the philosophy of at least one of these three schools. The work of Tantric scholar Douglas Brooks discussed next provides a foundation for understanding these three systems.

Classical Yoga

Classical yoga is the name given to those schools of yoga that consider themselves the most authentic representatives of Patanjali's *Yoga Sutras*. It is a dualistic philosophy that draws a clear distinction between the two major "substances" of the universe, *prakriti* (matter) and *purusha* (spirit). In Classical yoga matter and spirit are qualitatively different realities that never mix or join together. Spirit is absolute, unchanging, and superior to matter. Matter is relative, changeable, and inferior to spirit.

The essential nature of human beings is pure spirit, while everything in the physical world, including emotions and thoughts, is considered material. Human suffering is the result of confusing one's true nature with this lesser, material reality. The goal of Classical yoga is to separate these two realities, to extract one's true nature from the body/mind. It is designed to help students experience their immortal spirits. The goal of the yoga practice is to get into the body so you can get out of it. Sometimes these practices include harsh discipline that requires students to push beyond the pain in order to realize that they are something other than their bodies or their feelings. Because the body is inferior, it must be disciplined into submission so that spirit may be realized. If you are in a yoga class with a Classical yoga influence there will likely be a strong emphasis on controlling the body and mind through discipline. You may hear phrases like "push through the pain" when the postures become especially challenging.

For the Classical yogi the body and this physical life are problems to be solved. Birth is the result of a failure to realize our true nature in a previous life, and we are sentenced to come back again and again until we realize the truth. Freedom from the prison of embodiment comes when the seeker isolates the experience of pure spirit from the lesser realities of body, mind, and thoughts.

Advaita Vedanta

Vedanta means "conclusion or end of the *Vedas,*" because this method is based on the last set of Vedic texts and teachings, the *Upanishads*. In contrast to the dualistic philosophy of Classical yoga, *Advaita* (nondual) Vedanta negates the concept of separate realities for matter and spirit. In Advaita Vedanta only spirit is real; matter is an illusion. Our experience of matter, our bodies, our thoughts and feelings, and embodied life itself are an error in perception that can be corrected. There is only one true reality, but it appears as many to the unenlightened mind. This reality is unchanging and constant. Anything that changes, therefore, must be unreal. Since there is only one reality, all difference, as we perceive it in our worldly experience, simply does not exist. If we have a favorite flavor of ice cream or color of the rainbow it is simply an error of judgment. No perceived differences are real. All human suffering comes from this error of perception.

For Vedantins, like Classical yogis, this embodied life is a problem to be solved. And the Vedantins, too, have a solution. One of the primary strategies for overcoming erroneous thinking is referred to as *neti, neti* (not this, not this). The practice is to repeat phrases like "I am not my body, for my body changes," "I am not my mind, for my mind changes," "I am not my emotions, for my emotions change." Disciplined application of this approach is designed to bring true knowledge that will dispel the error in thought. Once the seeker acquires true knowledge, he or she becomes enlightened. An enlightened one may continue to inhabit the body but will have the awareness that the body, thoughts, and everything seen are just illusions. If you are in a hatha yoga class with an Advaita Vedanta influence you may hear phrases like "you are not your body" or "you are not your thoughts."

Tantra

Sometime around the fifth or sixth century B.C.E. there was another revolution in Indian philosophical thought regarding the nature of the universe and our relationship to it. It was a radical shift that gave rise to a body of texts, oral traditions, and practices known by the name *Tantra,* meaning "loom" or "weave" (also called *agama,* meaning "testimony").

Rather than join the argument between Classical and Advaita Vedanta yoga concerning the nature of matter and spirit, the Tantras transmuted it by agreeing with both sides and adding a new twist. Like Classical yogis, the Tantras affirmed the existence of spirit and matter; however, neither was granted supremacy. Like Advaita Vedantans, they affirmed the supreme unity of all reality. How could this be? How could both of the previously dominant philosophies be true at the same time?

Tantric philosophers resolved the issue with a masterful weaving together of these two great teachings. In essence they chose radical acceptance of all reality, both spiritual and material. The physical universe is explained as a diverse manifestation of the one supreme reality of divinity. The grounding matrix of physical reality (*prakriti* to Classical yogis) is the Vedantic supreme self. The world we live in is the manifestation of infinite forms of this supreme consciousness.

This was an incredible shift in the prevailing views, which considered the physical body as a problem to be solved and required self-denial and intense discipline of the physical body in order to either rise above it (Classical) or realize it as illusion (Advaita Vedanta). In bold contrast, the followers of Tantric philosophy considered the body as a manifestation of divinity itself, worthy of celebration and honor, rather than the result of a mistake or failure from a previous lifetime. This viewpoint was nothing less than a radical acceptance of the body and all of life as divinity incarnate. Suddenly there was nothing to renounce and no failed past life causing one's current birth, only the choice of living fully in the reality one has received as a divine gift.

In contrast to the Classical and Advaita Vedanta adherents who renounced the world as inferior or illusion, the followers of this new path were primarily lay people. They were heads of households and businessmen living in the everyday world,

Eight Limbs of Classical Yoga

As outlined earlier, the Classical yoga viewpoint follows a strict interpretation of the *Yoga Sutras*—the culmination of a long development of the science of yoga that set forth a very specific path to enlightenment. There are eight component stages, collectively referred to as *Ashtanga yoga* (*ashta,* "eight" and *anga* "limb"), the eight-limbed path to mystical union. The stages begin with a set of ethical codes and progress through physical postures, breathing exercises, and mental practices, culminating in the highest stage of absorption in the absolute.

Here is a description of the eight limbs:

1. *Yama*. Five virtues, or restraints, that govern our relationships with others and the world: *ahimsa* (noninjury), *satya* (truthfulness), *asteya* (nonstealing), *brahmacharya* (Godlike conduct), and *aparigraha* (nonclinging).

2. *Niyama*. Five observances of one's own physical appearance, actions, words, and thoughts that govern our relationship with ourselves: *shauca* (purity or cleanliness), *santosha* (contentment), *tapas* (heat, burning desire for reunion with God), *svadyaya* (self-study or self-inquiry) and *isvara pranidhana* (devotion or surrender to the Lord, "thy will be done").

3. *Asana*. Postures for creating firmness of body, steadiness of intelligence, and benevolence of spirit. The physical practice most familiar to Westerners as yoga.

4. *Pranayama*. A set of breathing exercises designed to help the yogi master the life force.

5. *Pratyahara*. Withdrawal of the senses, mind, and consciousness from the outside world; focus inward on the self.

6. *Dharana*. Focused concentration. With the body tempered by asanas, the mind refined by the fire of *pranayama,* and the senses under control using *pratyahara,* the student reaches this sixth stage.

7. *Dhyana*. Meditation. Withdrawing the consciousness into the soul.

8. *Samadhi*. Ecstasy. Merging with the divine. Self-realization. One experiences consciousness, truth, and unutterable joy. One must experience samadhi in order to understand it, because it is beyond the mind.

The system of Classical yoga based on the *Yoga Sutras* has undoubtedly been the most common style of yoga taught in the West. It holds a strong appeal for students who want a well-defined, stepwise approach to their spiritual advancement.

earning their living and paying their bills. Tantric scholar Douglas Brooks has coined the term *rajanakas* to refer to this group. The term *rajanaka* means "sovereign over one's own life"; it indicates that these yogis used their practice to gain mastery over all aspects of their lives while still living in the secular world. The modern day hatha yoga school called anusara yoga, founded by John Friend, is based on the Rajanaka Tantra tradition and draws upon the rich Tantric philosophy without the use of ancient Tantric ritual.

Needless to say, this fundamental shift toward Tantric thought affected the yogic practices of the day and continues to highlight the differences in the prevailing hatha yoga systems in the West. If you enter a yoga class based on Rajanaka Tantra philosophy you will likely hear phrases like "open to grace," "your body is a divine temple" and "shine out from your heart and express the divinity within you."

Paths of Yoga

Just as there are distinct philosophies and interpretations of the scriptures in world religions, different philosophies have formed in the world of yoga. Accordingly, the living science of yoga has been organized into many different paths or approaches over the centuries. It is no surprise that human beings, with so much diversity of thought and feeling, would find so many paths to their spiritual development in the realm of yoga. Yet, like many different paths to the top of the same mountain, all paths lead to the same goal. Many people find that, as they progress through their lives, more than one path speaks to their spiritual needs. The best yoga paths for you are simply the ones that appeal most to your heart.

There are a number of recognized paths of yoga, of which six have gained prominence in the Hindu culture of India: *bhakti, jnana, karma, raja, mantra,* and *hatha.*

Bhakti yoga is the yoga of devotion. It emphasizes the opening of the heart to divine love, the union of lover (the yogi) and beloved (the divine). This devotional love is often translated into song or chanting, with ecstatic repetition of the names of the beloved, in gatherings called *kirtans.* One of the most popular kirtan artists in the United States today is Krishna Das, who is a bhakti yoga practitioner.

Jnana yoga is the yoga of wisdom. *Jnana* means "knowledge." This is a path of self-realization through the exercise of discerning the real from the unreal or illusory. It is a practice of discriminating between the products of nature and the transcendental Self, until the true Self is realized in the moment of liberation. This is a strictly nondualistic (*Advaita Vedanta*) path that requires the seeker to separate the real from the unreal, the Self from the non-Self. Since the mind is considered part of the unreal, one must use the mind to outwit the mind. The principle techniques of this path are meditation and contemplation.

Karma yoga is the yoga of selfless action. *Karma* means "action." The karma yogi makes all actions an offering to God, with no thought of personal gain. Through serving others one is selflessly serving God. Mother Theresa and Mahatma Gandhi are examples of karma yoga practitioners.

Raja yoga is the "royal" yoga. *Raj* means "king," and raja yoga seeks to reveal the king within each of us that is normally hidden by our everyday actions and concealed by the workings of the mind. Raja yoga is a Classical yoga path most often associated with Ashtanga, the eight-limbed path of Patanjali. For the raja yogi the *Sutras* serve as an instruction manual to one's own experience of reality.

Mantra yoga is the yoga of sound. The word *mantra* comes from the root *man*, "to think" and the suffix *tra*, "suggesting instrumentality." So a mantra is a thought or intention expressed as sound. A mantra is a sacred utterance or sound charged with psychospiritual power. Yogis use mantras to achieve deep states of meditation and to invoke specific states of consciousness, and they believe that a mantra expressing a particular aspect of the divine will help to awaken that aspect of their own consciousness. For instance, a mantra to Ganesha, the remover of obstacles, is used to help awaken that part of our personalities that can overcome the obstacles in our lives. The most recognized and important mantra is the sound *OM* (see page 23).

Hatha yoga is called the forceful yoga and is defined in previous sections. There are many schools of hatha yoga, each rooted in one of the major philosophical traditions mentioned earlier (Classical, Advaita Vedanta, or Tantra). Many styles of hatha yoga have become popular in the West ranging from healing therapy to vigorous athletic flow. Some schools work with detailed physical alignment while others focus only on the inner experience. You may practice yoga in air-conditioned comfort or in temperatures of 100-plus degrees Farenheit (38+ °C). There is no shortage of variety and you are sure to find a style that agrees with you. Several styles of hatha yoga are listed in the resources section at the end of the book with contact information including websites where you can go to learn more about most of these styles.

Energetic Anatomy: The Chakras

The practices of yoga are designed to deal with our bodies on more than just a physical level. To the yogi the physical body is a manifestation, a reflection, of the astral or energy body. This body of energy has its own anatomy, based on seven major energy vortices called *chakras.* The word *chakra* means wheel or disk. The chakras line up along a central energy channel, or *nadi,* which runs from the base of the spine through the top of the head. It is called the *sushumna.* The sushumna is the energy body's primary pathway for the life force (*kundalini*). The chakras are nodes of connection along this pathway where other energy channels intersect. The goal of classical yoga is to awaken the kundalini energy that lies dormant at the base of the spine and make it rise to the highest energy vortex at the crown of the head. The Tantric approach is to stir one's awareness of that divine energy which is already awake. The yogi who can achieve and maintain this state is considered enlightened.

There are approximately 72,000 nadis in the energy body that channel energy. Three are primary, including the central sushumna and two others on either side. The left-side channel is called the *ida*. Its qualities are cool, soft, reflective, and sensitive, like the moon. The right-side channel is called the *pingala* and is associated with heat, activity, and strength, like the sun. The balance of energy flow on these two sides affects the sensations of heat and cold in the physical body. These two channels originate in the sushumna, near the base of the spine (in an energy vortex, or bulb, called a *kanda*), and they correspond to the first chakra, *muladhara*. They spiral up the sushumna, crisscrossing at each of the six higher chakras.

The chakras can be visualized from the front of the body as lotus flowers with the roots in the back. As the life force, or *prana,* moves through the system, it makes the chakras spin. The health of this system of energy flow depends on the chakras spinning at a proper speed. If the chakras spin too slowly, too weakly, or too fast, this creates a damming effect for the energy flow, and the system becomes imbalanced, which can manifest as emotional and physical illness.

Each chakra has a physical location in the body and is associated with physical, emotional, and energetic characteristics. Additionally, each chakra is associated with basic human rights and how we feel physically and energetically. For instance, if a child knows that he is loved, honored, and respected by his parents, he can develop a healthy sense of security. As a result the functioning of his muladhara chakra, which is associated with security, is enhanced.

The chakras can serve as a type of energetic health monitor for the student of yoga. As we perform the physical practice of hatha yoga we increase the health, awareness, and energy flow to each section of our bodies. If a particular section of our body is functioning at optimal levels energetically, the chakra associated with that section will also function optimally. Therefore, a hatha yoga practice can be designed to increase a student's self-esteem by strengthening the "band of self esteem," the region of the manipura chakra (the waistline).

Energy Gates: The Bandhas

Bandhas are a series of energy gates in the subtle energy body that regulate the flow of psychosomatic energy. The word *bandha* means lock, or constriction. You can think of the bandhas like the one-way valves in your circulatory system. These valves allow blood to flow in one direction as the heart pumps but not to reverse its flow on the upstroke, ensuring proper direction of blood flow. The bandhas direct the life force in a similar way.

Yoga practitioners learn to tone certain sets of muscles in order to provide a lock, or closure, that holds psychosomatic energy and moves it powerfully through the subtle energy channels. This generates a psychic heat in the subtle body that helps to stimulate the awakening of the kundalini energy.

There are three primary bandhas in the body:

Mulabandha—the root lock—is located at the base of the spine. It stops the downward flow of life force, *apana*, so that it can be equalized with the upward flow, *prana*. The physical location of mulabandha is the perineum (the soft tissue between the anus and the genitals). *Mulabandha* comes as you draw energy through the muscles of the perineum toward a central point, creating an energetic lift through the core of the body. It is often difficult for beginners to access these muscles until they have increased their body awareness in this area. Such awareness can be increased by engaging the pelvic floor muscles as you would to stop the flow of urination. With heightened awareness mulabandha can be practiced by drawing energy through the muscles of the perineum toward a central point, creating an energetic lift through the core of the body.

Uddiyana bandha. *Uddiyana* means "flying upward." This "gate" is located in the low abdomen. Uddiyana bandha is performed by exhaling fully and drawing the lower abdomen in and up while simultaneously lifting the diaphragm. It is important not to engage this bandha after eating or during deep inhalation, as it puts pressure on the stomach, lungs, and other internal organs. This bandha is intended to create further lift for the upward flow of prana in the sushumna.

Jalandhara bandha—chin or throat lock—is located at the top of the throat. This lock stops prana flow from leaking upward out of the torso and downward from the head into the torso. *Jala* means "net," "web," or "mesh." This lock is performed as follows: While lengthening your neck, curl your head back initiating the movement from the palate as if drinking sweet nectar. Keeping your neck extending upward, release your head forward like the bow of a swan, taking the top of your throat back and up as if your throat were smiling from ear to ear. Continue the release of your chin toward your chest while taking the top of the throat back and up.

Performed together, these bandhas create an energy container between the floor of the pelvis and the throat chakra. The psychic heat generated helps to mobilize the upward rising of the kundalini energy and clear blockages in the central energy channel.

When you attend a hatha yoga class you may be taught how to use the bandhas by the specific names referred above. Or you may not hear the word bandha mentioned at all. Some schools of hatha yoga teach bandhas most of the time, while others teach them sparingly but some schools use alignment principles to create the same effect.

This book follows the latter approach for teaching asanas. *Mulabandha* is engaged by the following sequence of instructions which are common to many asanas in this book—move your thighs back; widen your pelvic floor; keeping that action, tuck your tailbone down and under; and extend from your low belly up through the top of your head. *Uddiyana bandha* is engaged by the following instructions—draw the flesh below your navel in and up (take the sides of your waistline back) and extend from your low belly up through the top of your head. Techniques for *jalandhara bandha* are not explored in this book.

Using Drishtis

A *drishti* is a gaze, or a point of focus. Drishtis are included for each pose in chapters 2 through 10 of this book as a way to direct your focus when you practice. Dristhis are actually intended to direct your "inner" focus more than your physical sight, even though the directions may be to fix your gaze on an external object or a point on your body, such as the floor, the tip of your nose, or your navel. Dristhis are designed to help you practice your yoga with awareness and without being distracted by your surroundings. Use them to practice the postures in this book if you find them helpful.

Getting the Most From Your Yoga Practice

Now that you have been exposed to some of the history and philosophy of yoga, let's introduce some of the basic elements to consider in your yoga practice. Simple choices you make about clothing, time, your place of practice, and the use of props can make all the difference in your enjoyment and make the time you spend practicing yoga most effective. Learning how to use your breath during yoga is highly important to enhance your practice and make your practice the best it can be for you. You will likely find that meditation is a wonderful complement to your practice of yoga and an equally powerful stand-alone practice that you will enjoy for years to come. All of these practices will be introduced in the sections that follow so that your yoga toolbox will be well stocked when you begin your practice of hatha yoga.

Yogic Breathing

Our breath is synonymous with our life. Breathing is so natural and automatic that most people never even notice that they are breathing unless it is excited or restricted in some way. Life enters us with our first inhalation and leaves with our final exhalation. It is truly one with our life force. The animating life force of the breath can be thought of as the play of a divine goddess, called *Shakti*. Shakti is the creative energy of the divine that animates everything in the universe. In essence we are always being breathed by this divine energy. When we inhale the Shakti is exhaling into us, and when we exhale it is her inhale.

For the yogi the breath serves as an extension of the prana, or life force, as it moves in the body. It is the physical manifestation of the natural flow of this energy. It is the medium through which we express the attitude in our hearts and translate it into the outer body. By using the breath we increase our sensitivity to the flow of energy, and with that increased sensitivity we are closer to realization of our own divine nature. The breath has the capacity to open the body and allow our energy to flow more freely in our yoga practice. Awareness of breath brings a mindful, sacred quality to an asana practice.

One of the first lessons to learn in the practice of yoga is proper use of the breath. Yoga is a practice of connecting to the deep spirit within each of us. It is the practice of tuning in to the essence of our hearts, all of our dreams and desires, and expressing them joyfully through our physical bodies. The breath is the medium through which we make that connection.

> The breath interweaves the threads of one's intentions into the fibers of the outer body. It is the uniting force between mind and body— heart essence and outer vessel.
>
> **John Friend, founder of Anusara Yoga, *Anusara Yoga Teacher Training Manual***

The Natural Breath

When we are born, our breath is full, flowing, and uninhibited. Our bodies and minds are designed for the fullest expression of the breath. We don't have to think in order to breathe in that way. This type of breath just happens with no conscious effort on our parts. Anusara Yoga founder John Friend calls this type of breathing "the natural breath" for which he identifies several key characteristics:

1. The pelvic floor expands and descends on inhalation and contracts and lifts on exhalation.

2. The collarbone lifts and rolls upward on inhalation and descends on exhalation.

3. The upper arms externally rotate on inhalation and internally rotate on exhalation.

You can see this process most clearly in the breathing of a baby, whose belly will rise and fall with each breath. Babies seem to breathe with their whole bodies, as if every part expands and contracts with the movement of the breath. You can observe your own diaphragmatic breathing by lying on your back and noticing the natural rise and fall of your belly with the breath.

The natural breath wants to flow in us as the fullest possible expression of the Shakti energy. However, if mental or emotional traumas are introduced we may learn different breathing habits that restrict this natural flow. For instance, when we are threatened or upset our whole body tightens we enter a state commonly referred to as the fight-or-flight response. In such a state we are reduced to our basic survival instincts—the abdomen tightens, restricting diaphragmatic breathing, and quick, shallow chest breathing results. This state might be healthy for a person who has stepped in front of a bus. However, chronic exposure to circumstances that elicit the fight-or-flight response can cause a person to form long-term restricted breathing habits. The emotional stresses of a fast-paced lifestyle can cause a person to lose touch with the fullness of his or her breath. It is not uncommon for Westerners to use only a small percentage of our breathing capacity. Returning to an awareness of our natural breath can help us to recover our healthy breathing patterns.

Uninhibited breathing creates the natural rise and fall of the belly because of the movement of the diaphragm, the main muscle responsible for breathing. The torso of our bodies is divided into two main cavities—the thoracic, or chest cavity, and the abdominal cavity. At the bottom of our chest cavity we have a muscular membrane called the diaphragm, which completely separates these two cavities. Like the head of a drum stretched across the bottom of our rib cage, the outline of the diaphragm is roughly the outline along the base of the ribs. It attaches to the bottom of the sternum (the center chest, where the ribs attach) and follows the lowest outline of the ribs all the way back to the lumbar spine, where it attaches via tendinous tissues called crura. There are three openings in the "drum head" of the diaphragm to allow descending and ascending blood to flow and food to pass. The heart rests just above the diaphragm, and the digestive organs are just below it. The lower surfaces of the lungs are attached to the upper surface of the diaphragm.

As the diaphragm moves through a large range of motion it substantially changes the volume of the thoracic cavity. The muscles of the rib cage and upper chest also change thoracic volume, although with much less efficiency than the diaphragm.

When we breathe naturally the diaphragm moves down to create a vacuum in the chest cavity that draws the air into the lungs. Because the downward movement of the diaphragm displaces the organs of the abdomen, the belly naturally distends on inhalation and retracts on exhalation as in the natural breath. You can increase your awareness of your diaphragm by placing a small, soft weight, such as a bag of rice or beans, on your abdomen between your ribs and your navel. As you inhale, notice the work that the diaphragm must do to lift the extra weight. As you exhale, let your belly gently fall under the weight. Simply increasing your awareness of your natural breath, without trying to manipulate or control your breathing, can bring you to a state of peace and relaxation.

Diaphragmatic Breathing

A yogic practice that consciously uses the diaphragm with the breath is called *diaphragmatic* breathing. The following exercise is a remedial form of diaphragmatic breathing that helps to counter those problems that interfere with the natural breath.

Begin the exercise in a reclining position with your spine resting on a stack of blankets. Fold three firm-weave blankets (Mexican blankets work well) lengthwise to a width just less than the width of your shoulders and to a length just longer than the distance from your navel to the top of your head. Stack two of the blankets one on top of the other. Stack the third blanket crosswise to the other two at one end of the stack. Sit on the floor in front of the stack, and lie back with your head resting on the third blanket such that your head is slightly elevated. From this position you can easily practice breathing into the three regions of your torso, as follows:

Lower belly: Place your hands on your low belly, just above the navel, with the tips of your middle fingers touching. Breath with your diaphragm so that your belly rises into your hands and your fingertips separate slightly. Also allow the breath to fill the side and back belly region so that there is a full expansion in all directions. As you exhale allow the lower torso to contract so that your fingers come back into contact. Practice several breaths in and out of the low-belly region of your torso.

Mid-chest: Place your hands on the sides of your rib cage and apply a slight inward pressure to your ribs. As you inhale, in addition to lifting the low belly, consciously expand the sides of your rib cage to make more room for the breath. Notice how the ribs both expand into your hands and separate slightly from each other. Continue this breathing practice for several breaths.

Upper chest: Place your hands on your upper chest with your index fingers resting on your collarbones. Breathe into your hands by filling your upper chest with your breath and notice the expansion upward into your hands. You will notice the least amount of movement into this region even as the amount of effort is substantially greater.

Full Yogic Breathing

The next step in a yogic breathing practice is to learn *full yogic breathing.* This technique also uses all three areas of the torso to allow the fullest breath possible with two significant changes from diaphragmatic breathing: 1) With full yogic breathing as you inhale, you tone the muscles of your low abdomen so that your torso expands to the side with your breath rather than having your belly rise; 2) on exhalation, you keep your ribs expanded (as if you are inhaling).

To practice full yogic breathing in the reclining position repeat the three steps described for diaphragmatic breathing within the duration of a single breath. On inhalation keep the low belly toned so that your belly does not rise. As you exhale, keep your chest expanded and full and empty the air from top to bottom. Keep your breath smooth and steady, and attempt to make the duration of the inhalation and exhalation the same. You may discontinue placing your hands on your torso once you have learned the technique. Once you've mastered this breathing in the reclining position, you may attempt it in a sitting position. For this practice, keep your pelvis heavy on inhalation as you breathe into all three torso regions successively. On exhalation, keep your ribs lifted and expanded.

Other Breathing Techniques

Over the centuries yogis have understood the power of the breath to alter states of consciousness and have developed breathing techniques to create a desired state. These techniques of the breath are called *pranayama*.

It is interesting to consider the use and interpretation of these breathing techniques from the perspective of the major yogic schools. Some Classical yogis translate pranayama as "breath control," a combination of the Sanskrit terms *prana*, or life force (breath), and *yama*, "control" or "restriction." This interpretation makes sense from the Classical perspective that the body is inferior to spirit and is to be dominated or forced into submission so that we can realize our true nature. In another interpretation the body and the breath are seen as manifestations of divinity. Accordingly, pranayama is interpreted as *prana* and *ayama*, which means "noncontrol." From this perspective the techniques are seen as a way of skillfully participating with the breath, or dancing with the divine goddess Shakti.

There are a wide variety of breathing techniques that have been developed, depending on the desired state the yogi wishes to attain. Two of the most common pranayamas are described below.

Ujjayi Breathing   *Ujjayi,* which means "victoriously uprising," is the most common yogic breathing technique. You will hear the sound of *ujjayi* breathing in almost any yoga class. It is created by toning the epiglottis to intentionally create a sound at the back of your throat. The sound has been compared to the whispered sound of *haaa* in the back of your throat as you breathe. It creates a direct feedback that yogis use to monitor the flow of their breath. The quality of your breath is directly related to your state of mind, so when you are aware of your breath you can be aware of your inner state.

To practice *ujjayi* breathing take a deep inhalation followed by a deep exhalation, to open yourself up to receive the breath. Inhale through your nose as you slightly constrict the muscles in the back of your throat to create a whispering sound. Exhale through your nose creating the same sound. Keep the flow of your breath even and smooth from the beginning to the end of each inhalation-exhalation cycle. Generally we inhale and exhale faster at the beginning of the cycle, and our breath tapers off at the end. During *ujjayi*, keep the same rate of breath flowing at all times, from start to stop. This requires that you make the second half of each inhale or exhale stronger to balance the flow. Fill yourself with the breath from bottom to top as in full yogic breathing, creating lift in the spine and torso, and keep the lift as you exhale. Breathe smoothly and steadily, making your inhalation and exhalation even in duration. This type of breathing is very soothing to your nervous system and promotes calmness and peace of mind.

Alternate Nostril Breathing   This type of yogic breathing is called *nadi shodhana.* As described earlier the word *nadi* means "energy channel" and *shodhana* means "cleansing." Nadi shodhana breath is designed to cleanse the nadis. You will recall that there are three main channels in the body for prana: one central (sushumna), one right (pingala), and one left (ida). Usually there is a difference in the energy flow between the right and left channels that shifts back and forth during the day. You can notice this by the difference between your left and right nostrils as you breathe. One side will be dominant for a while, and then the pattern will reverse. The alternating breath of nadi shodhana both cleanses and balances the flow between ida and pingala.

Alternate nostril breathing requires a little technique for regulating the breath through one nostril at a time. To experience this technique hold out your right-hand palm, face up. Curl your index and middle fingers to touch the fleshy part of your palm at the base of your thumb. Keep your thumb extended and free (figure 1.1a). You will use your thumb to close off your right nostril and your other two fingers to close off your left nostril.

The technique for nadi shodhana is as follows:

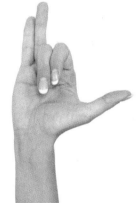

Figure 1.1a

1 Put your right hand into the form just described. Begin with a deep inhalation.

2 Close your left nostril with your ring finger and exhale fully through your right nostril (figure 1.1b).

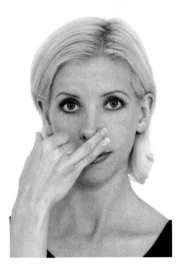

Figure 1.1b

3 Inhale fully through your right nostril, close your right nostril (using your thumb) as well, and pause (figure 1.1c).

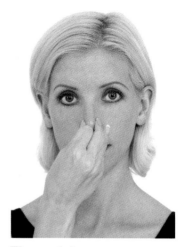

4 Open your left nostril, exhale fully through the left side, and pause (figure 1.1d).

Figure 1.1c

5 Inhale fully through your left nostril, close your left nostril as well, and pause. Open your right nostril and exhale fully through the right side.

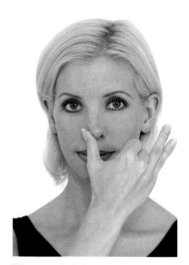

6 Repeat this pattern for a few minutes, then finish with inhalation through your right nostril and exhalation through both nostrils. Return to natural breathing.

Figure 1.1d

What to Wear

When you practice hatha yoga the most important thing about clothing is that it be comfortable and functional. Your clothing should not restrict your movements and should be appropriate for the temperature of the room in which you practice. It is essential to remove socks and shoes when practicing yoga so that your feet will stick to your yoga mat (see the next section "How to Use Props") and your feet and toes will be able to expand.

For public yoga classes that use alignment principles, such as Anusara Yoga or Iyengar Yoga, it is important to wear clothing that allows your teacher to see your alignment. For instance, long, baggy pants do not allow the teacher to see if your leg muscles are properly engaged or if your knees are properly aligned. And if you are trying to learn to properly engage your shoulder blades on your back you will need visibility there. For these classes tights and leotards are recommended for women, shorts and tank tops for men. For classes that do not emphasize alignment, you can have fun wearing the latest in yoga apparel to class. For restorative and gentle classes the more comfortable you are, the better. In general, your clothing should support your practice, be comfortable, and be fun.

How to Use Props

The most important piece of equipment you will need to start your yoga practice is a good yoga mat. A yoga mat provides a nonslip surface that will keep you steady as you move into and out of various postures. There are many different types of mats available. It is best to choose a good-quality mat that supports your practice. The thinnest mats (about 1/8 inch thick) are rubberized, colorful, and provide a good nonslip surface; however, these mats do not provide much cushion for bony protrusions when you are doing floor exercises. The thickest mats are called *transformer mats*. These mats provide excellent cushion and nonslip characteristics though they are quite heavy and expensive. It is a good idea to use the mats your yoga studio provides for a while until you decide what type is best suited for you.

There is a variety of other props that will support your practice as well. A good yoga blanket is a must for the beginning student. Most studios provide blankets so that you do not have to purchase your own. The best blankets are of the Mexican close-weave variety. These fold with crisp, clean edges and provide the most stable support. Synthetic, loose-weave blankets or towels do not provide stable support.

Yoga blocks, straps, bolsters, sandbags, and eye pillows are also useful props when called for by your teacher or in the asana descriptions. Most studios provide all of the props for no charge except mats, which can usually be rented for a small fee per class. Eye pillows are usually purchased separately.

Yoga blankets placed under your hips provide extra cushion and lift to help you keep your low back from rounding when you're sitting on the floor. Straps provide extra reach when you are extending your legs and reaching for your toes as well as support for some sitting and partner postures. Yoga blocks can be placed under your hands in side and forward bends until you can reach the floor without them. Blocks can also be squeezed between your thighs in some postures to teach proper engagement of the legs. Sandbags provide weight for extra grounding for floor exercises. They can encourage relaxation when placed on your body because they give a safe, stable pressure. Eye pillows are very calming for restorative postures and final relaxation. They provide a gentle, even pressure on your eyelids.

Where to Practice

The great thing about your yoga practice is that it is truly portable. You may decide to practice yoga at places and times other than just public classes. If you are away from home, and depending on the level of your practice, you may decide to practice in an airport during a layover (headstands are great conversation starters), in a hotel room (after moving the furniture), or at work in a vacant conference room.

You may want to create a special space in your home for your practice. A room with a hardwood floor or smooth tile is ideal. A low-pile carpet can also make a good surface for yoga practice if you use a good yoga mat to help you avoid slipping. Yoga mats are now widely available in locations ranging from yoga studios to grocery stores.

When to Practice

The most important aspect of when you choose to practice is that you are regular and consistent in your practice. The more you practice yoga the more you will progress. Allow yourself one or two days off per week to give your body time to recover, as needed. If you are menstruating or ill be willing to take a few days off for that as well. In general it is best to commit to practicing daily for a set amount of time, even if you cannot practice at the same time each day. Choose a time that fits your schedule when you will not be distracted by other things. Figure out how much time you can give to your yoga practice each day. Even if you practice as little as 15 to 20 minutes a day you will notice improvements in your strength and flexibility and in the way you feel. As you progress you can add to your practice time in preparation for a full-length public class (typically 90 minutes long).

If you practice in the morning you may notice that your mind is keen but your body is a little sluggish. In the late afternoon or early evening your body is usually flexible but your mind may be tired and lacking focus. The body and mind are usually at their peak in the late morning and early afternoon, so those are optimal times for a full asana practice. There are many studios and class times available in most cities and towns, so you should be able to find a time that works for you.

You should not practice yoga when you have a fever. Yoga raises the body temperature and competes for the energy your body needs to recover. Likewise, do not practice if you are weak from cold or flu, except to do restorative postures. Women should avoid doing inversions such as headstand or shoulder stand when they are menstruating. This is because the healthy downward flow of the menses is disrupted if a woman inverts during this time. A woman can substitute a supported Downward-Facing Dog or Legs-Up-the-Wall pose in this case.

Always seek the advice of your physician and your yoga instructor about practicing if you are ill or injured. A yoga instructor who is skilled in the art of yoga therapy can help you greatly if you are injured. But be sure that your teacher has been properly trained in yoga therapy. The two schools of hatha yoga that are most respected for yoga therapy are Anusara Yoga and Iyengar Yoga.

When you are ready to attend public yoga classes, it is recommended that you attend at least twice weekly in order to progress in your practice. This book provides excellent training to prepare you for your first class and can remain an outstanding reference for you as you progress in public classes and deepen your own home practice.

What and When to Eat

There are a few general guidelines to follow for eating before yoga practice, such as finish meals three to four hours before an intense practice. It is best if the digestive process is complete before you practice yoga, because digestive muscles compete with other body muscles for blood after you eat. If you have low blood sugar or have little time between yoga sessions for a meal you can supplement with fruit, energy bars, or yogurt anywhere from 30 to 60 minutes before class. Protein smoothies also make an excellent quick meal when time is short, because liquids are more easily digested.

For some schools of hatha yoga the issue of vegetarianism is a serious concern, while for others it hardly receives mention. Disagreements on the morality of what we eat can result in heated confrontations within and outside of the yoga community. For most of us the way we eat is a deeply personal issue. For many it is also an issue of how we treat the other beings on our planet.

Arguments against a diet including meat are usually based upon the concept of *ahimsa* from Patanjali's *Yoga Sutras.* There are many levels of interpretation of this principle. Some define ahimsa as nonviolence and take the stance that taking any form of life to further your own is a violent act. Some yoga practitioners go so far as to wear masks and sweep the ground in front of them to avoid taking the lives of insects.

Others interpret ahimsa as noninjury and view the world as inherently containing acts of violence, such as cutting the umbilical cord on a baby or defending your self or loved ones from attack. If violence cannot be avoided in an engaged life, the injury it does can be skillfully managed. For this school of thought it is not the act itself that is important, it is the intent behind the act. The main measure of an act is whether or not it is *shri,* or life-affirming. For example, chemotherapy is a very violent act against the body, yet the intent is to save the life of the patient.

For others the choice of how to eat is primarily a matter of health and happiness. Certain types of diet are healthier than others and directly affect the quality of your life. It is beyond the scope of this book to offer detailed dietary advice. Most people who practice yoga find that they are more aware of how their bodies feel and how their diet affects their bodies. As we increase our sensitivity to the gift of our body we are likely to move naturally toward the best choice for ourselves.

Learning to Meditate

Meditation is the basis for all inner work. It is the direct naked encounter with our own awareness that shifts our understanding of who we are and gives us the power to stand firmly in our own center. No one else can do this for us. Only meditation can unlock these doors.

Swami Durgananda (Sally Kempton), *The Heart of Meditation*

Meditation is an important part of the journey inward. It is a gateway into your experience of your own inner nature of divinity. Many great yogis have followed the pathway of union with the self through meditation. A strong and supple body greatly enhances your experience of sitting meditation. Many Westerners are not aware that the postures of hatha yoga were originally created to prepare the body for sitting meditation.

Patanjali's *Yoga Sutras* call for meditation, or *dhyana*, as the seventh stage of the eight-stage path to enlightenment. Once students have mastered the sixth stage (concentration, or *dharana*), they may proceed to meditation. But almost everyone begins their meditation practice while they are still working to increase their ability to concentrate, so do not be discouraged as you observe your mind wandering. That is normal.

The dictionary defines meditation as a devotional exercise of contemplation. The root Latin word for meditation, *meditari*, means "to think about or consider." Any form of contemplation can be a meditation if you are focused clearly on the issue at hand. For instance, time you spend considering how you want to live and who you want to be in this life are excellent examples of meditation. Even if you are confused about your course of action, meditation can connect you to your heart, where there is a deep knowing about the right choices. The more you meditate, the more you will learn to trust your own inner source of guidance.

It is not necessary to meditate if you practice hatha yoga. Nor is it a requirement to practice yoga if you want to meditate, but combining the two practices can enhance your experience of both.

Ways to Meditate

There are many ways to meditate, just as there are many styles of yoga. The best way to determine the best style of meditation for yourself is simply to try several styles and see which one says *yes* to your heart.

The first stage of meditation is to focus clearly on a specific object or sensation with your eyes open or closed. You can repeat a word or phrase, visualize a place, object, or deity, or simply tune in to your breath and observe it slowly coming in and going out.

Sound meditation usually involves the use of a mantra to draw you into deep states of awareness, as described in the "Paths of Yoga" section of this chapter. A mantra is a sacred utterance or sound charged with psychospiritual power. It is usually a word or phrase honoring a particular deity or aspect of the divine. Yogis use mantras to achieve deep states of meditation and to invoke specific states of consciousness, and they believe that a mantra expressing a particular aspect of the divine will help to awaken that aspect of their own consciousness. A mantra is used to help awaken that part of our personalities that can overcome the obstacles in our lives. The most recognized and important mantra is the sound *OM*. Silently repeating your chosen mantra as you sit in meditation can be very powerful.

The *OM* was considered the single most important sound in chanting of the *Vedas*. The symbol for *OM*, illustrated in figure 1.2, represents all the states of human consciousness and is interpreted as follows. The bottom curve represents the dream state, the upper curve represents the waking state, and the middle curve, or swirl, to the right represents the deep, dreamless sleep state. The crescent shape (top right) represents the veil of illusion, or *maya*, and the dot represents the transcendental state.

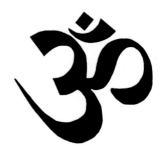

Figure 1.2 Symbol for *OM*.

For some people, visualization meditation may be more effective. You can visualize your chosen deity—a god or goddess or a peaceful nature scene, such as a flower or a beautiful coastline. The image you choose should elicit feelings of deep contentment for you.

Another popular meditation technique is simply to focus on your breath. There is no attempt to control or change the breath. Just focus on all aspects of your breathing—how your chest lifts and your abdomen expands and how the air feels moving through your nostrils. There is no judgment, no good or bad aspect of the breath, just awareness. The breath is a manifestation of the divine energy that animates your body. This meditation helps bring to consciousness the awareness that you are being breathed by that divinity.

Heart-centered meditation involves focusing on your heart center and the feelings and sensations that arise there. Focusing on our hearts takes us deeply into our core awareness and our most profound feelings of love and joy. You can visualize the breath moving directly into your heart center to begin to connect with these feelings.

Where to Meditate

> You must have a room, or a certain hour or so a day, where you don't know what was in the newspapers that morning, you don't know who your friends are, you don't know what you owe anybody, you don't know what anybody owes you. This is a place where you can simply experience and bring forth what you are and what you might be. This is the place of creative incubation.
>
> Joseph Campbell, *The Power of Myth*

The place you choose for your meditation is important. It is the way you honor both your meditation ritual and yourself. Select a sacred space to support your meditation practice in a way that honors the things that have meaning for you. You may choose a space filled with light and fresh air or one that is cozy and warm. The most important thing is that your space helps to transport you to that sacred place within yourself.

Also, it is powerful to come back to the same place each time you sit for meditation. Your continued practice will build the energy in your space, establishing a strong, peaceful vibration. The ideal space is a room with no other purpose (except possibly your hatha yoga practice). If it is not possible to set aside a whole room just for meditation, select a corner of a room that is free from distraction.

It is a wonderful practice to create an altar in your meditation space. An altar can transform your mediation space, because it creates a sense of ritual. And ritual can take you right into your heart, because it serves to remind you of what is important. Your altar can be anything you want it to be as long as it is something that matters to you. There are no rules, so be creative. Some items you might use on your altar are candles, incense, pictures of teachers or others you look up to, and pictures of deities or great beings. These items will uplift your senses and establish a pure energy. Flowers can be an offering to your favorite deities or can simply invite your heart to open.

When to Meditate

The best times to meditate are just before sunrise and at sunset. These are the times when nature slows her activity, birds are quiet, and animals do not stir. Because we are connected with the natural world our minds and bodies are also still at these times, yet we can remain alert. As often as possible, practice your meditation at the same time each day. Consistency builds a strong and useful meditation practice.

Your meditation practice can be an excellent complement for your asana practice. If you begin or end your practice with 5 to 10 minutes of meditation you will find that both practices benefit. However you do it, it is recommended that you create a regular meditation practice. Even 5 to 10 minutes each day will show positive results in your state and clarity of mind.

Positions for Meditation

The Classical position for meditation is sitting on the floor in a cross-legged position. The sitting positions are chosen because they allow the meditator to sit comfortably for relatively long periods. A common meditation asana that allows for extended sitting (20 to 90 minutes) are the sage positions (siddhasana), see page 176. If you are unable to sit in one of these positions, you can meditate sitting with good posture in a chair.

Proper alignment when you sit will help to make your experience more enjoyable and productive. To practice meditation sitting, refer to the photographs and instructions in chapter 9.

Begin your meditation by either practicing one of the techniques just described or a technique of your own choosing. It is a good idea to set a timer to let you know when your allotted time has passed to avoid the distraction of watching the clock.

Mudras

A *mudra* is a hand gesture, an asana for the hands. Throughout history, hand gestures have been used by all civilizations and religions. The priests and priestesses of ancient Egypt used hand gestures to perform prayer rituals 5,000 years ago. People of many cultures have used them, including the Aborigines, Romans, Turks, Persians, Africans, Chinese, Gigians, Mayans, and Native Americans. Christians will recognize specific hand gestures in the portrayals of Jesus, though few know the significance of these mudras. The most commonly recognized mudra is the "prayer" mudra, known to yogis as *anjali mudra*. Anjali means "offering"—this mudra can represent offering to one's self in service or in gratitude. In India mudras became very important with the practices of yoga.

The word *mudra* means "seal," because the mudras create an impression in the subtle body like a letter sealed with a hot-wax imprint. The impressions are made in the energy body and, therefore, are used to control the flow of life energy in the body. This life energy, or prana, radiates from the fingertips. Each finger conducts a different vibrational energy, and these finger postures bring the energies together in different combinations. Each combination completes an energy circuit in the body and mind, creating a calming effect that also stimulates various chakras. There are many combinations of finger postures to encourage different kinds of mental focus. Because of the effect on the chakras, mudras may also be helpful in healing various medical conditions. Kundalini yoga and other modalities use mudras for this purpose.

These are some of the most commonly known yoga mudras:

Adi mudra: *Adi* means "first," and adi mudra is the first position in which an infant holds its hands—making a fist with the thumb tucked inside. Adi mudra is used to control clavicular (upper-chest) breathing. It stimulates the deepest recesses of the brain, that organ which is most closely associated with the crown chakra.

Abhaya mudra: The "gesture of fearlessness" for dispelling fear in others. This mudra is shared and understood equally by Native Americans, Hindus, Buddhists, and the Christian painters of the Renaissance. When you raise your right hand, extending your fingers straight up and holding your palm open, you are showing peaceful and compassionate intent. This mudra relates to the anahata (heart) chakra.

Agni mudra: *Agni* means "fire," which in yoga is commonly associated with the digestive process. In agni mudra the thumb touches the tip of the middle finger; the first, third, and fourth fingers are extended away from the palm. Agni mudra improves both digestion and intelligence, and is good for the manipura (abdominal) chakra.

Apan mudra: Also known as the "deer mudra" because of the antlerlike pointing of the index and little fingers. *Apana* refers to the cleansing effect of prana when it flows down and out of the body. In this mudra the tip of the thumb contacts the tips of both the second and third fingers; the first and fourth fingers point upward like the antlers of a deer. It promotes a patient and serene state of mind.

Gyana mudra: This mudra is accomplished by touching the tip of the thumb and index fingers together. The second, third, and fourth fingers are extended away from the palm. This is the most popular mudra for meditation, as it promotes calmness and clarity of mind.

Dhyana mudra: *Dhyana* means "meditation." The hands are placed palms up in the lap, right on top of left, with the tips of the thumbs touching. Some of these mudras are used with the asanas in chapter 9.

Using the Asanas in This Book

The remainder of this book provides a step-by-step guide for how to perform a wide array of yoga poses or *asanas*. Each chapter contains similar asanas that are grouped according to type of posture, such as backbends, forward bends, balancing postures, and so forth. Each posture is listed by both English and Sanskrit names (when available) and most include a counterpose, which you may perform as a cool-down following the original pose, and a drishti, which you may use as a point of focus. The physical and mental benefits as well as the contraindications are listed to help you understand the benefits of each pose and any necessary variations or precautions for performing certain poses.

Each posture is presented as a series of photos with step-by-step instructions to help you get into and out of the pose. Many poses also include a gentle variation that can serve as a good starting point for beginners or that can provide an option for those with physical limitations. Finally, most asanas list variation postures that will provide greater challenge as your practice progresses.

This book can be used as an excellent reference for your practice of yoga whether you are a beginning, intermediate, or advanced practitioner. Each posture will open up to you the more you practice it and you may find that you can come back to the same posture again and again and learn something new each time. This book will serve as your own personal guide along your yoga adventure. Enjoy the journey.

chapter 2

Standing Postures

Standing postures are the most fundamental class of all asanas because they create the foundation for your practice by laying the groundwork for the more advanced postures. They help you increase power, strength, and stability in the legs. In addition, they aid in proper digestion, circulation, mobility, and spatial awareness. During a series of standing postures the heart and lungs actively detox the blood. Following standing postures, the nervous system is better insulated, therefore leaving you feeling refreshed, attentive, and settled.

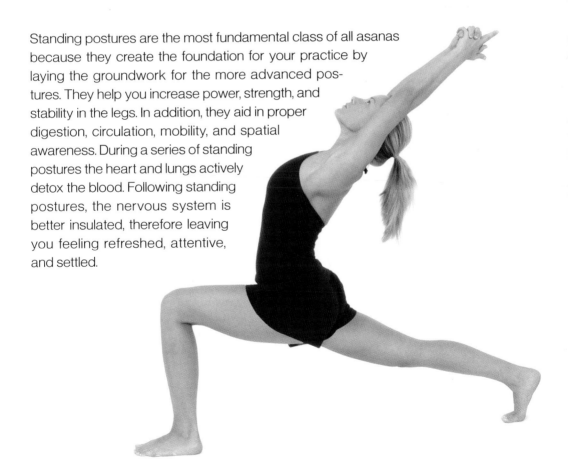

Mountain

Tadasana

Drishti

▷ Forward

Physical Benefits

▷ Aligns the spine
▷ Tones the abdominal muscles and buttocks
▷ Opens the chest
▷ Improves posture
▷ Strengthens the arches, ankles, knees, and thighs

Mental Benefits

▷ Improves focus
▷ Develops willpower
▷ Reduces mild anxiety

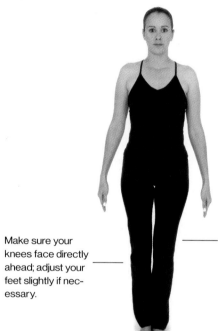

Make sure your knees face directly ahead; adjust your feet slightly if necessary.

Hug your leg muscles to the bone on all sides by engaging the muscles from skin to muscle and muscle to bone; pull the muscles up from your feet into your pelvis.

1 Stand with your feet parallel. Draw an imaginary line from the center of your ankle through the second toe of each foot and make those lines parallel to each other.

2 Inhale and take the tops of your thighs back so that your hips stick out in back. Exhale and balance the backward action of your thighs by lengthening from your tailbone downward through your feet. This action moves your hip flesh down and creates a lifting action below your navel. Inhale and extend from your pelvis up through the top of your head, keeping your heart lifted and your chest open.

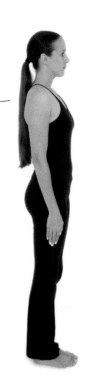

Lengthen the sides of your body, take your shoulders back, and bring the shoulder blades more onto your back.

3 Stay in the pose for several full breaths and notice how you feel, then release.

Other Variations

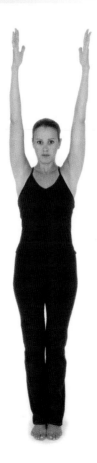 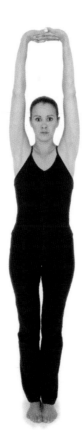 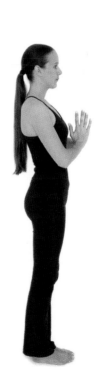

Downward-Facing Dog

Adho Mukha Svanasana

Counterpose
▶ Child's Pose (Balasana)

Drishti
▶ At the floor
▶ Between your feet

Physical Benefits
▶ Improves digestion
▶ Relieves insomnia, menstrual and menopausal discomfort, and low back pain
▶ Strengthens the arms, legs, and torso
▶ Stretches the palms, chest, back, hamstrings, calves, and feet
▶ Energizes the body

Mental Benefits
▶ Improves focus
▶ Develops willpower
▶ Stimulates the mind
▶ Relieves stress and mild anxiety

Contraindications
▶ Carpal tunnel syndrome
▶ High blood pressure
▶ Headache

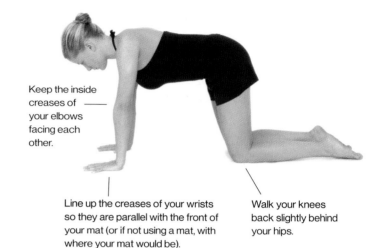

Keep the inside creases of your elbows facing each other.

Line up the creases of your wrists so they are parallel with the front of your mat (or if not using a mat, with where your mat would be).

Walk your knees back slightly behind your hips.

1 Come to all fours, placing your hands directly under your shoulders. Spread your fingers evenly and root down into the floor through all four corners of your hands. Rooting down means to extend downward energetically like a tree sending down roots into the earth. Inhale and draw muscularly from your hands up into your shoulders. Keeping your arms steadfast and straight, exhale and draw your shoulder blades onto your back.

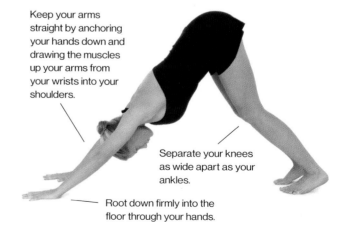

Keep your arms straight by anchoring your hands down and drawing the muscles up your arms from your wrists into your shoulders.

Separate your knees as wide apart as your ankles.

Root down firmly into the floor through your hands.

2 Maintaining the action of step 1, inhale, lift your hips, and lengthen back through your spine and hips.

3 Straighten your legs to come into the full pose.

Lengthen from your heart down through your arms and up to your tailbone.

Press your thigh bones back into your hamstrings.

4 Hold for a few breaths. Release and lower yourself into Child's Pose.

Keeping the toes spreading, root from your tailbone down through your legs to bring your heels toward the floor.

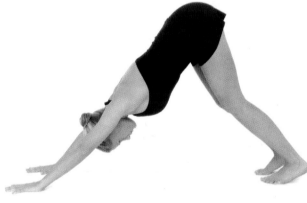

Gentle Variation

Follow steps 1 through 3 except keep your knees bent and your heels off the floor.

Other Variation

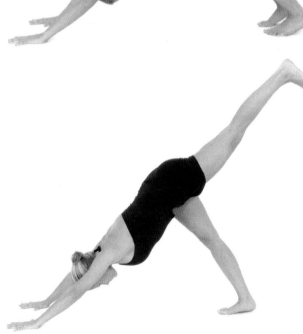

Extended Side-Angle

Utthita Parsvakonasana

Counterpose
- Downward-Facing Dog (Adho Mukha Svanasana)

Drishti
- Upward
- Forward
- At the floor

Physical Benefits
- Strengthens the ankles, calves, knees, and thighs
- Relieves symptoms of sciatica
- Opens the hips and groin
- Increases lung capacity
- Alleviates symptoms of arthritis
- Lengthens the spine
- Improves digestion

Mental Benefits
- Builds focus
- Develops willpower
- Stimulates the mind
- Reduces stress

Contraindications
- Knee injury
- Low blood pressure (keep fingertips upward, toward the ceiling)

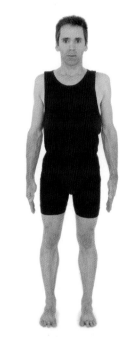

1 Stand in Tadasana (see page 28).

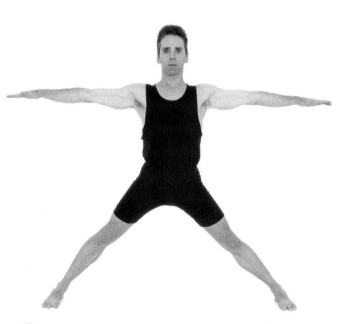

2 Step your feet wide apart. Inhale and extend your arms out to the side. Ideally your ankles should be under your wrists.

3 Turn your left foot in slightly and turn your right leg out directly to the side.

4 Exhale, bend your right knee to 90 degrees, and place your right fingertips on the outside edge of your right ankle. Place your left hand on your hip. Take your hips and thighs back, widen your sitting bones apart, and widen the pelvic floor. Keep the space between your sitting bones and root your tailbone down, extending from your pelvis down through your feet. Extend your left arm over your left ear and look up under the arm.

5 Hold for several breaths, then pull your legs toward each other, inhale, and come up. Repeat on the other side.

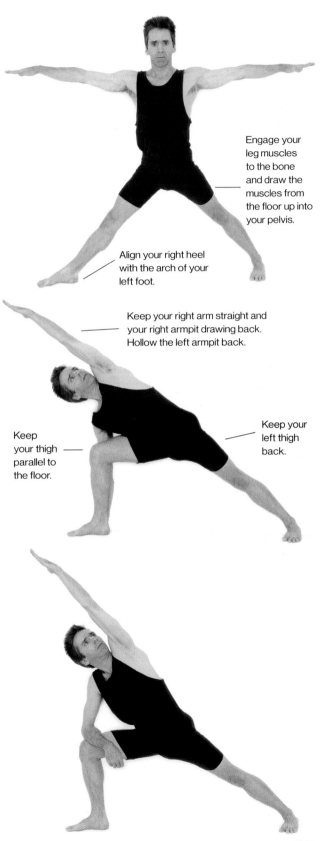

Engage your leg muscles to the bone and draw the muscles from the floor up into your pelvis.

Align your right heel with the arch of your left foot.

Keep your right arm straight and your right armpit drawing back. Hollow the left armpit back.

Keep your thigh parallel to the floor.

Keep your left thigh back.

Gentle Variation

Follow steps 1 through 5 except rest your elbow on your knee rather than taking the fingers to the floor.

Triangle

Utthita Trikonasana

Counterpose
- Standing Forward Bend (Uttanasana)

Drishti
- Upward
- Forward
- Down

Physical Benefits
- Improves digestion and circulation
- Helps relieve menopausal discomfort
- Relieves symptoms of sciatica
- Stretches the arches, calves, hamstrings, and groin
- Opens the throat, chest, shoulders and hips
- Lengthens the spine
- Stabilizes and strengthens the legs and torso
- Increases muscular endurance

Mental Benefits
- Builds focus
- Develops willpower
- Stimulates the mind
- Relieves stress

Contraindications
- Neck injury (do not look up)
- Low blood pressure
- Congestive heart disorders

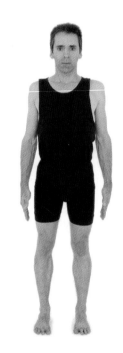

1 Stand in Tadasana (see page 28).

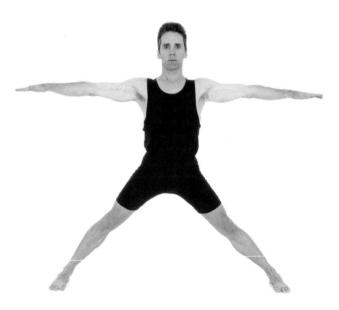

2 Step your feet wide apart. Inhale and extend your arms out to the side. Ideally your ankles should be under your wrists.

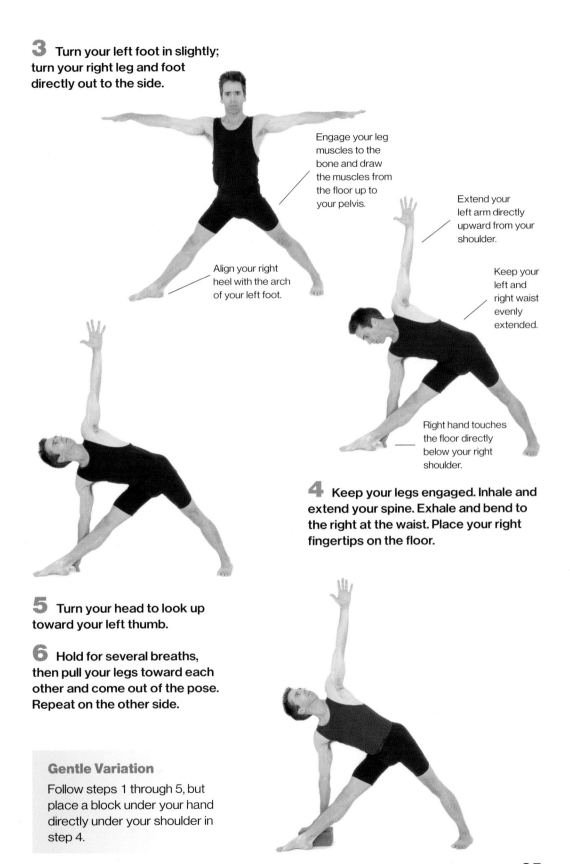

3 Turn your left foot in slightly; turn your right leg and foot directly out to the side.

Engage your leg muscles to the bone and draw the muscles from the floor up to your pelvis.

Align your right heel with the arch of your left foot.

Extend your left arm directly upward from your shoulder.

Keep your left and right waist evenly extended.

Right hand touches the floor directly below your right shoulder.

4 Keep your legs engaged. Inhale and extend your spine. Exhale and bend to the right at the waist. Place your right fingertips on the floor.

5 Turn your head to look up toward your left thumb.

6 Hold for several breaths, then pull your legs toward each other and come out of the pose. Repeat on the other side.

Gentle Variation

Follow steps 1 through 5, but place a block under your hand directly under your shoulder in step 4.

Warrior II

Virabhadrasana II

Counterpose
▷ Downward-Facing Dog (Adho Mukha Svanasana)

Drishti
▷ Over fingertips of forward extended hand

Physical Benefits
▷ Strengthens the arches, ankles, knees, and thighs
▷ Stretches the hips and shoulders
▷ Broadens the chest
▷ Increases lung capacity
▷ Stimulates digestion and circulation
▷ Enhances muscular endurance
▷ Lengthens the spine

Mental Benefits
▷ Builds focus
▷ Develops willpower
▷ Stimulates the mind

Contraindications
▷ High blood pressure
▷ Neck injury

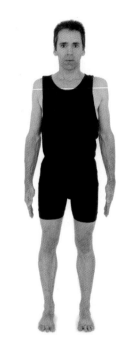

1 Stand in Tadasana (see page 28).

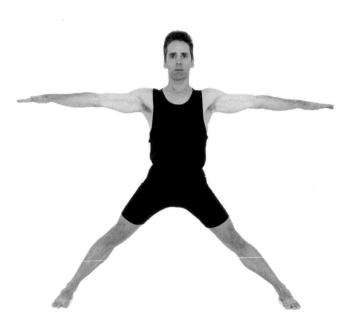

2 Step your feet wide apart. Inhale and extend your arms out to the side.

3 Turn your left foot in slightly; turn your right leg out directly to the side.

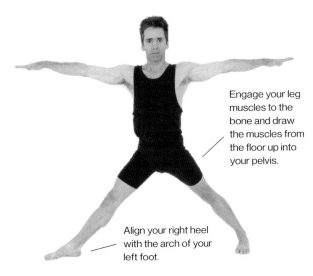

Engage your leg muscles to the bone and draw the muscles from the floor up into your pelvis.

Align your right heel with the arch of your left foot.

4 Keeping your legs engaged, exhale and bend your right knee to 90 degrees.

5 Hold for several breaths. To release, pull your legs toward each other to engage the muscles, inhale, and come out of the pose. Repeat on the other side.

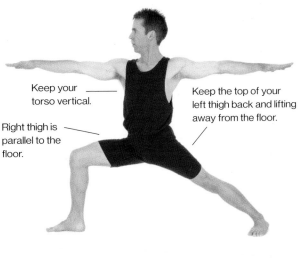

Keep your torso vertical.

Right thigh is parallel to the floor.

Keep the top of your left thigh back and lifting away from the floor.

Other Variation

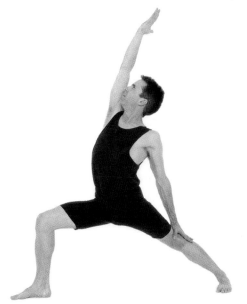

Crescent Lunge

Alanasana

Counterpose
▷ Downward-Facing Dog
(Adho Mukha Svanasana)

Drishti
▷ Forward
▷ Upward, through fingertips

Physical Benefits
▷ Strengthens the arches, ankles, knees, and thighs
▷ Stretches the hips and shoulders
▷ Opens the chest
▷ Stimulates digestion
▷ Increases muscular endurance
▷ Relieves symptoms of sciatica

Mental Benefits
▷ Builds mental focus
▷ Develops willpower
▷ Stimulates the mind

Contraindications
▷ Neck injury
▷ Knee injury (use the gentle variation)

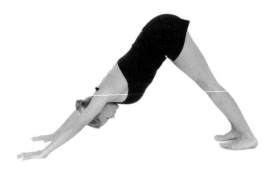

1 Start in Downward-Facing Dog (see page 30).

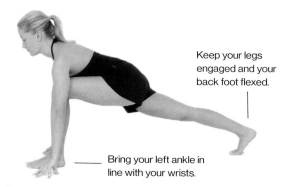

Keep your legs engaged and your back foot flexed.

Bring your left ankle in line with your wrists.

2 Inhale, step your left foot forward into a lunge, and keep your back leg straight.

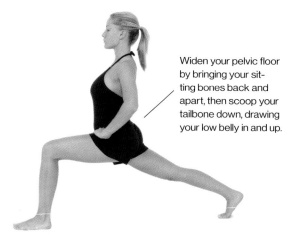

Widen your pelvic floor by bringing your sitting bones back and apart, then scoop your tailbone down, drawing your low belly in and up.

3 Inhale and lift your torso up and bring your hands onto your hips. Press down with your left foot and pull it back against the resistance of the floor as you pull from the right foot forward to square your hips.

38

4 Inhale and stretch your arms over your head and clasp your hands with the index fingers pointing up to the ceiling. Exhale and root from your low belly down through your feet. Inhale and extend from your low belly up through your hands. Lengthen your neck and press your head back to curl your shoulder blades more onto your back in a back bend. Hold for a few breaths. Pull your legs toward each other as in step 3, inhale, and come up. Repeat on the other side.

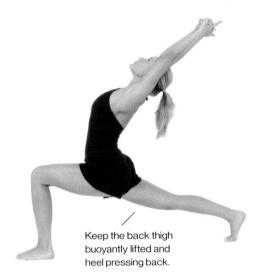

Keep the back thigh buoyantly lifted and heel pressing back.

Gentle Variation

Follow steps 1 through 4 except keep your back knee on the floor and your hands unclasped shoulder-width apart.

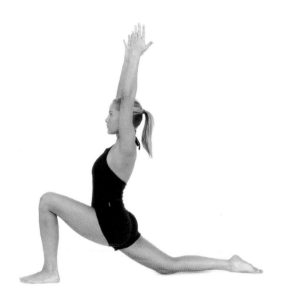

Other Variation

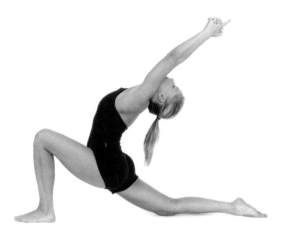

Warrior I

Virabhadrasana I

Counterpose
- Downward-Facing Dog
  (Adho Mukha Svanasana)

Drishti
- Forward
- Upward

Physical Benefits
- Strengthens the arches, ankles, knees, and thighs
- Stretches the hips and shoulders
- Broadens the chest
- Stimulates digestion and circulation
- Increases muscular endurance
- Relieves symptoms of sciatica

Mental Benefits
- Builds focus
- Develops willpower
- Stimulates the mind

Contraindications
- High blood pressure
- Neck injury

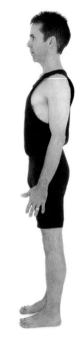

1 Stand in Tadasana (page 28).

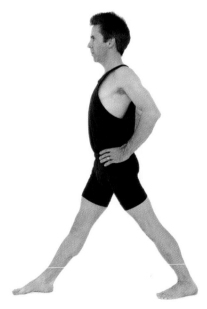

2 Step your right foot forward one full, comfortable stride. Turn the heel of your left foot in slightly so that the foot faces out at a slight angle.

3 Keeping your legs engaged, exhale and bend your right knee to 90 degrees. Place your hands on your hips and square them to the front. Adjust the distance between your feet as needed so that your right shin is perpendicular to the floor when your right thigh is parallel to the floor. Inhale and extend your arms over your head. Root your tailbone down, extending from your pelvis down through your legs.

Keep your arms straight by squeezing your triceps and lengthening up through your fingertips.

Keep your fingers open and draw muscularly from fingertips down into the shoulder socket.

Extend from your pelvis up through the crown of your head.

Keep your right knee directly over your ankle.

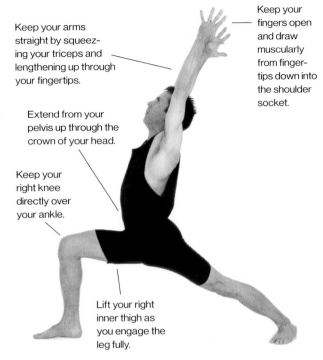

Lift your right inner thigh as you engage the leg fully.

4 Hold for a few breaths. To release, root down through your feet into the floor, inhale, straighten your front leg, and come up to standing. Repeat on the other side.

Revolved Extended Side-Angle

Parivrtta Parsvakonasana

Counterpose

▷ Standing Forward Bend
(Uttanasana)

Drishti

▷ Upward

▷ Forward

▷ At the floor

Physical Benefits

▷ Strengthens the ankles,
calves, knees, and thighs

▷ Relieves symptoms of
sciatica

▷ Opens the hips and groins

▷ Increases lung capacity

▷ Alleviates symptoms of
arthritis

▷ Lengthens the spine

▷ Improves digestion

▷ Improves balance

▷ Stimulates the circulatory
and lymphatic systems

Mental Benefits

▷ Builds focus

▷ Develops willpower

▷ Stimulates the mind

▷ Reduces stress

Contraindications

▷ Knee injury

▷ Low blood pressure

▷ Migraine

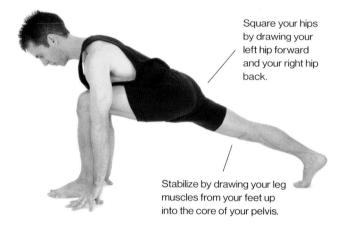

Square your hips
by drawing your
left hip forward
and your right hip
back.

Stabilize by drawing your leg
muscles from your feet up
into the core of your pelvis.

1 **Start in a Lunge with your left foot forward
and your right leg straight.**

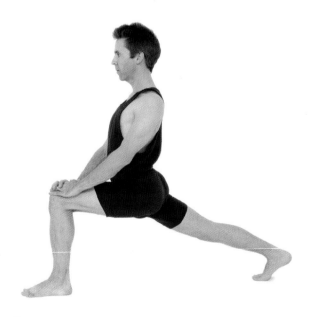

2 **Keeping your legs engaged, lift your torso and
place your hands on your front thigh.**

3 Keep your legs hugging in to stabilize your pelvis, and use your hands against your left thigh to twist your torso to the left.

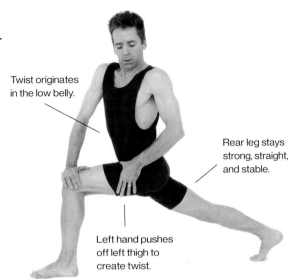

Twist originates in the low belly.

Rear leg stays strong, straight, and stable.

Left hand pushes off left thigh to create twist.

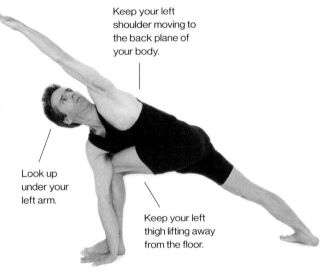

Keep your left shoulder moving to the back plane of your body.

4 Hook your right armpit as deeply as possible across your left knee and place your right hand on the floor. Spin your right leg so that the foot is flat on the floor. Extend your left arm over your left ear, palm face down.

Look up under your left arm.

Keep your left thigh lifting away from the floor.

5 Hold for several breaths, then pull your legs toward each other and come out of the pose. Repeat on the other side.

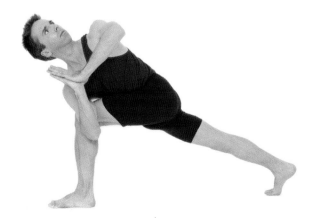

Gentle Variation

Follow steps 1 through 4, then press your palms together in a prayer position. Drop the back knee if necessary.

Revolved Triangle

Parivrtta Trikonasana

Counterpose
- Standing Forward Bend (Uttanasana)

Drishti
- Upward
- Forward
- At the floor

Physical Benefits
- Improves digestion and circulation
- Tones and stretches the calf, thigh, hamstring, and abdominal muscles
- Lengthens the spine
- Opens the throat, chest, and shoulders
- Strengthens the hip muscles and opens the groin
- Improves balance

Mental Benefits
- Builds focus
- Develops willpower
- Stimulates the mind
- Relieves stress and mild anxiety

Contraindications
- Migraine
- Insomnia
- Low blood pressure

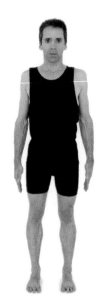

1 Stand in Tadasana (page 28).

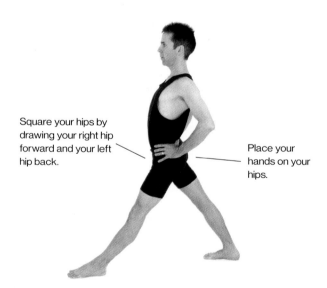

Square your hips by drawing your right hip forward and your left hip back.

Place your hands on your hips.

2 Step your left foot 3 to 3 ½ feet forward and turn your right foot out at a slight angle. If you are unable to square your hips, step your right foot to the right a few inches until you can bring the hips in line.

3 Inhale and lengthen from your pelvis up through your head. Exhale, bend forward, and place your fingertips on the floor.

4 Bring your left hand to your hip. Inhale and extend from the core of the pelvis out through the crown of the head, lengthening the spine. Exhale and twist your torso to the left, starting from your low belly. Then twist your ribs, shoulders, and head, in that order, and raise your left arm to the ceiling.

5 Hold for several breaths, then place your left hand on your hip and turn your gaze to the floor. Bring your right hand up to your other hip. Lengthen your spine from the core of your pelvis out through the crown of your head. Root down through your feet into the floor, inhale, and come up. Repeat on the other side.

Gentle Variation

Follow steps 1 through 5, but place a block under your hand in step 4.

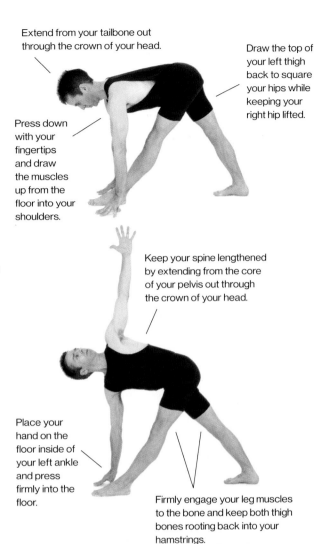

Extend from your tailbone out through the crown of your head.

Draw the top of your left thigh back to square your hips while keeping your right hip lifted.

Press down with your fingertips and draw the muscles up from the floor into your shoulders.

Keep your spine lengthened by extending from the core of your pelvis out through the crown of your head.

Place your hand on the floor inside of your left ankle and press firmly into the floor.

Firmly engage your leg muscles to the bone and keep both thigh bones rooting back into your hamstrings.

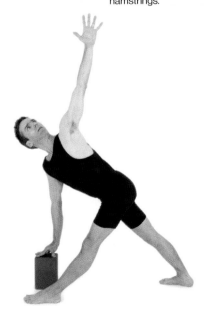

Chair

Utkatasana

Counterpose
▶ Standing Forward Bend (Uttanasana)

Drishti
▶ Forward
▶ Upward

Physical Benefits
▶ Lengthens the spine
▶ Strengthens the feet, ankles, calves, knees, buttocks and thighs
▶ Opens the chest
▶ Stimulates the digestive, circulatory and reproductive systems

Mental Benefits
▶ Builds focus
▶ Develops willpower
▶ Stimulates the mind
▶ Reduces stress

Contraindications
▶ Low blood pressure
▶ Insomnia
▶ Knee injury (use the gentle variation)

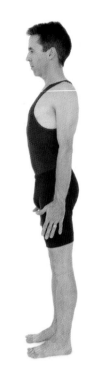

1 Stand in Tadasana (page 28).

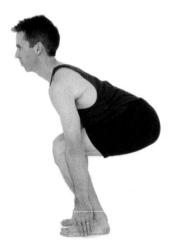

2 Exhale, bend your knees to 90 degrees, and touch your fingertips to the floor.

3 Inhale and stretch your arms overhead. Draw from your fingertips down into the shoulder sockets

4 Hold for 15 to 30 seconds. To release, inhale, straighten your legs, and stand up. Exhale and lower your arms to your sides.

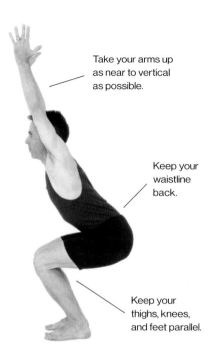

Take your arms up as near to vertical as possible.

Keep your waistline back.

Keep your thighs, knees, and feet parallel.

Gentle Variation

Follow the steps 1 through 3 except bend the knees only slightly and remain in the pose for a few breaths.

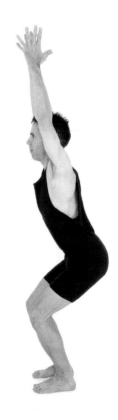

Standing Intense Spread-Leg Pose

Prasarita Padottanasana

Counterpose
▷ Standing Forward Bend (Uttanasana)

Drishti
▷ At the floor
▷ Eyes closed
▷ Tip of nose

Physical Benefits
▷ Strengthens the feet, ankles, knees, inner thighs, and lower back
▷ Improves digestion and circulation
▷ Tones abdominal cavity
▷ Reduces minor backache
▷ Relieves headache and symptoms of sinusitis

Mental Benefits
▷ Builds focus
▷ Develops willpower
▷ Calms the mind
▷ Reduces stress and anxiety

Contraindications
▷ Low back injury (use the gentle variation)
▷ High blood pressure

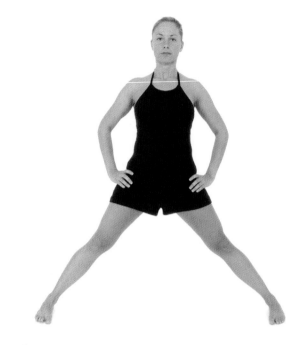

1 Stand with your legs 4 ½ to 5 feet apart and your feet parallel. Place your hands on your hips. Inhale and extend from your pelvis up through your head.

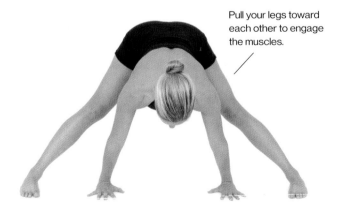

Pull your legs toward each other to engage the muscles.

2 Exhale, bend forward, and place your hands on the floor with your fingertips in line with your toes.

3 **Exhale and bring the top of the head to the floor.**

Exhale, root your tailbone down and extend from your pelvis through your feet. Inhale and extend from your pelvis out through the crown of your head.

Draw your shoulder blades onto your back.

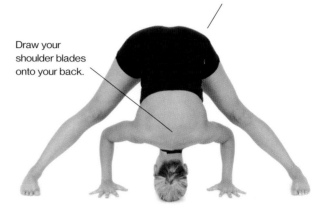

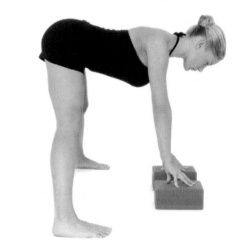

Gentle Variation

Follow steps 1 and 2, but place a block directly under each shoulder for your hands.

Other Variation

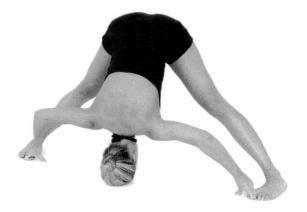

Beam

Parighasana

Counterpose

- Child's Pose (Balasana)

Drishti

- Forward
- Upward

Physical Benefits

- Lengthens the side of the body
- Opens the chest
- Tones the abdominal organs
- Strengthens the ankle, knee, and hip joints
- Stretches the arches, calf, thigh, and abdominal muscles

Mental Benefits

- Increases clarity
- Reduces stress

Contraindications

- High blood pressure—keep both hands above heart level
- Sciatica
- Hip, knee, or groin injury

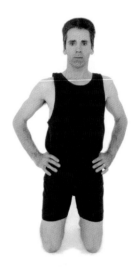

1 Kneel on the floor with your hands on your hips and flex your feet.

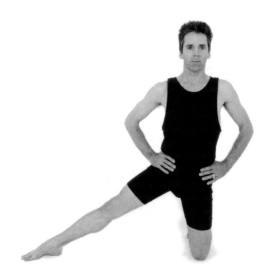

2 Stretch your right leg out to the side and keep your foot in line with your left knee. Turn your right foot in at an angle.

3 Inhale and stretch your arms out to the sides, parallel with the floor.

Engage the band of muscle above your right knee to keep your leg straight.

Lengthen up through the sides of your body.

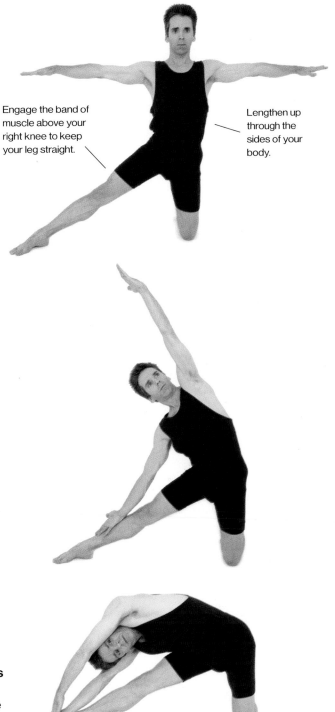

4 Inhale and draw muscularly from your right foot up into the core of your pelvis. Take the sides of your waistline back, lengthen your tailbone down, round your back, and bring your torso slightly forward. Exhale, bend your torso to the right, and slide your right hand down your leg, palm facing up. Bring your left arm over by the side of your ear.

5 Keep your back rounded, exhale, stretch your right arm over to the left, and touch your palms together. Stay for a few breaths. To release, pull your legs toward each other, inhale, and return to standing. Repeat on the other side.

Gentle Variation
Follow steps 1 through 4 only.

Humble Warrior

Counterposes

- Standing Forward Bend (Uttanasana)
- Downward-Facing Dog (Adho Mukha Svanasana)

Drishti

- Forward
- At the floor

Physical Benefits

- Stretches the sides of the body
- Opens the chest
- Tones the abdominal organs
- Strengthens the ankle, knee, and hip joints
- Opens the hips
- Stimulates the thyroid and parathyroid glands
- Lengthens the spine
- Helps alleviate symptoms of carpal tunnel syndrome in wrists and forearms
- Improves balance
- Strengthens the thighs, calves, and feet

Mental Benefits

- Increases clarity
- Reduces stress, mild depression, and anxiety

Contraindications

- Low blood pressure—keep your head above your heart
- Knee injury
- Pregnancy (after the first trimester)

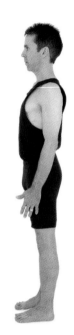

1 Stand in Tadasana (see page 28) with your feet parallel and hip-width apart.

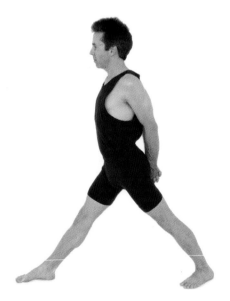

2 Bring your legs wide apart. Turn your left foot in, turn your right foot out, and turn your torso to the right. Square your hips and clasp your hands together.

3 Inhale, lengthen up through the sides of your body, pin the heads of your arm bones back, and draw your shoulder blades onto your back. Exhale, bend your right knee, and extend your torso over your right leg.

Extend from the core of your pelvis out through the crown of your head.

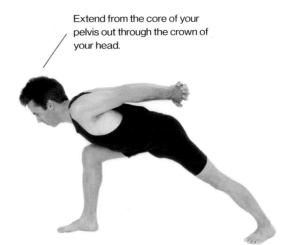

4 Exhale, bend your torso forward between your legs, and bring your head close to the floor.

5 To release, pull your legs toward each other. Inhale and return to standing. Repeat on the other side.

Keep your shoulder blades engaged on your back and draw your arms up toward the ceiling.

Engage the band of muscle above your left leg to maintain the straightness.

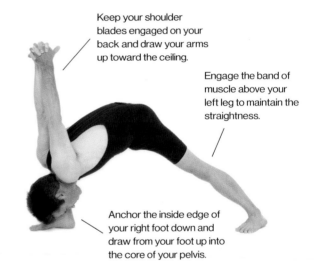

Anchor the inside edge of your right foot down and draw from your foot up into the core of your pelvis.

Gentle Variation
Perform a Lunge with your back knee down.

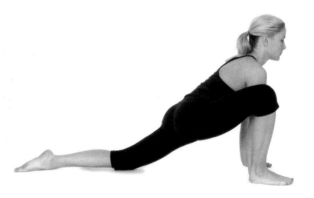

Intense Side-Stretch

Parsvottanasana

Counterpose
▷ Standing Forward Bend
(Uttanasana)

Drishti
▷ Upward
▷ Forward, on shins

Physical Benefits
▷ Opens the chest
▷ Strengthens the feet,
ankles, shins, knees, and
thighs
▷ Releases the hips
▷ Stretches the hamstrings
▷ Improves digestion and
circulation
▷ Stimulates the thyroid and
parathyroid glands
▷ Tones the abdominal
muscles
▷ Lengthens the spine
▷ Improves balance

Mental Benefits
▷ Increases clarity
▷ Reduces stress

Contraindications
▷ Low blood pressure
▷ Pregnancy

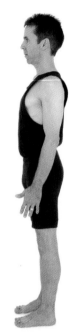

1 Stand in Tadasana (see page 28) with your
feet parallel and hip-width apart.

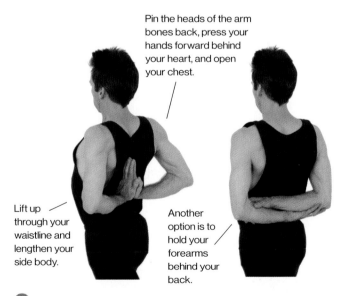

Pin the heads of the arm
bones back, press your
hands forward behind
your heart, and open
your chest.

Lift up
through your
waistline and
lengthen your
side body.

Another
option is to
hold your
forearms
behind your
back.

2 Inhale and bend your elbows and join your
palms together behind your back with the fingers
pointing up. Exhale and slide your folded hands up
your back between your shoulder blades.

3 Exhale, step your right foot forward 3 to 3½ feet, and square your hips.

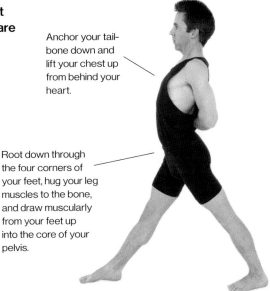

Anchor your tailbone down and lift your chest up from behind your heart.

Root down through the four corners of your feet, hug your leg muscles to the bone, and draw muscularly from your feet up into the core of your pelvis.

4 Maintain the extension of your spine. Exhale and bend your torso forward.

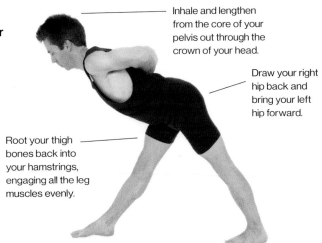

Inhale and lengthen from the core of your pelvis out through the crown of your head.

Draw your right hip back and bring your left hip forward.

Root your thigh bones back into your hamstrings, engaging all the leg muscles evenly.

5 Continuing your exhalation, extend your torso forward over your leg and bring your chin to the top of your shin. Stay in this pose for several breaths. To release, hug your legs together (pull them toward each other) and root down through your feet into the floor. Inhale and return to standing. Repeat on the other side.

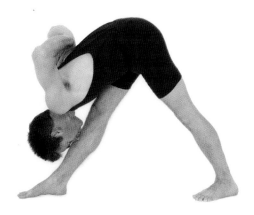

Gentle Variation

Follow steps 1 through 4, keeping your hands on your hips. Use blocks under your hands for the final step.

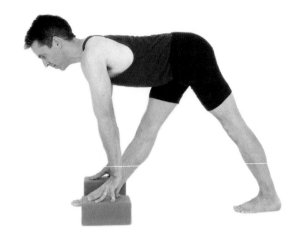

Other Variations

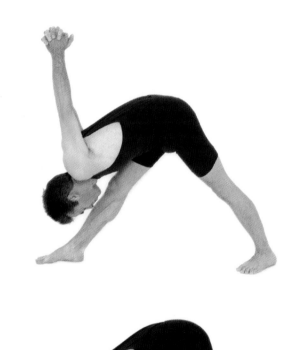

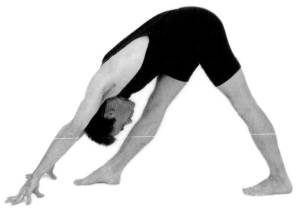

chapter 3

Balancing Postures

Balancing postures require a great deal of focus, strength, and stamina. They develop poise, agility, coordination, and concentration. They require you to draw into your core muscles and thus, your inner awareness. They are strengthening poses in which muscle tone is created and precise alignment is essential. Regular practice of the balancing postures shown in this chapter helps you develop increased control over your body.

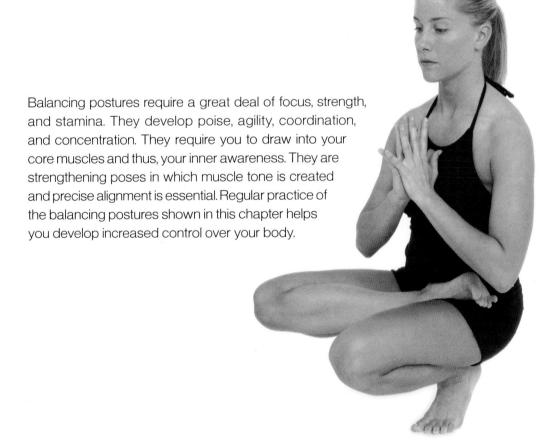

Eagle

Garudasana

Counterpose
▶ Mountain (Tadasana)

Drishti
▶ Forward

Physical Benefits
▶ Improves balance
▶ Strengthens the feet, ankles, calves, and thighs
▶ Opens the shoulders, chest, back, and hips
▶ Improves digestion and circulation
▶ Stimulates the pituitary and thyroid glands

Mental Benefits
▶ Builds focus
▶ Develops willpower
▶ Stimulates the mind

Contraindication
▶ Knee injury

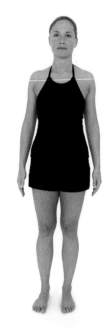

1 Stand in Tadasana (see page 28).

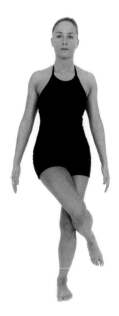

2 Balance on your left leg with your knee slightly bent. Lift your right leg and cross it over your left leg at the knee.

3 Hook your right foot behind your left shin, hugging your legs together.

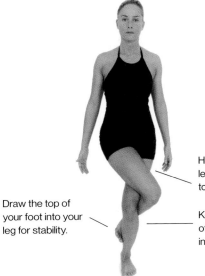

Draw the top of your foot into your leg for stability.

Hug your legs together.

Keep the knee of your standing leg bent.

Lift your elbows and extend from your elbows through your fingers.

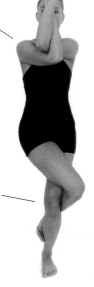

4 Cross your left elbow over your right and join the palms of your hands.

Squeeze the muscles of the standing leg on all sides.

5 Hold for several breaths, come out of the pose and repeat on the other side.

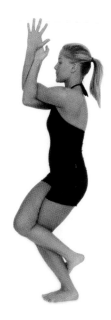

Tree

Vrksasana

Counterpose
▷ Standing Forward Bend
(Uttanasana)

Drishti
▷ Forward
▷ Upward

Physical Benefits
▷ Remedies flat feet
▷ Strengthens the arches,
ankles, calves, and thighs
▷ Lengthens the spine
▷ Improves balance
▷ Opens the shoulders, chest,
thighs, and hips
▷ Improves circulation

Mental Benefits
▷ Calms the mind
▷ Cultivates poise and focus

Contraindications
▷ Headache
▷ High blood pressure (keep
hands under the heart)

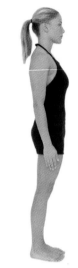

1 Stand in Tadasana (see page 28).

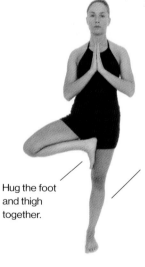

Hug the foot
and thigh
together.

Take the tops of
your left thigh back,
lengthen your tail-
bone down, and
extend from the
core of your pelvis
through your left leg
into the ground.

2 Spread your toes and root down through all
four corners of your feet. Inhale and draw muscularly from your feet up into the core of the pelvis
and hug your legs together. Focus on a point in
front of you. Keeping your left leg strong and
steady, inhale, bend your right leg and place the
right foot against the inner left thigh. Bring your
palms together in front of your heart.

3 Inhale, lengthen the sides of your body from the hips up to the shoulders and bring your shoulder blades onto your back. Extend your arms over your head beside your ears and bring your palms together.

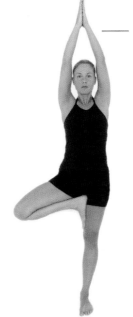

Keep the arms fully engaged and straight.

4 Hold for several breaths then lower the arms and leg simultaneously. Repeat on the other side.

Gentle Variation

Follow the instructions for steps 1 and 2, but bring your foot only as high as your ankle.

Other Variation

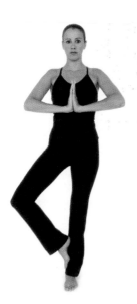

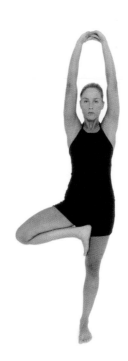

Tiptoe Pose

Counterpose
- Standing Forward Bend (Uttanasana)

Drishti
- At fingertips
- Forward
- Eyes closed

Physical Benefits
- Strengthens the arches, ankles, calves, and thighs
- Lengthens the spine
- Improves balance
- Relieves symptoms of sciatica
- Opens the shoulders, chest, thighs, and hips
- Improves digestion and circulation

Mental Benefits
- Builds focus
- Develops willpower
- Calms the mind
- Cultivates poise

Contraindications
- Headache
- Low blood pressure
- High blood pressure

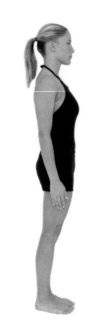

1 Stand in Tadasana (see page 28).

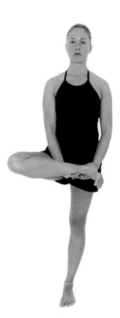

2 Balance on your left leg. Bend your right knee, hold your right foot, and draw your knee out to the side. Take your heel up toward your navel.

3 Roll your right foot and leg forward and down, and place your foot at the left thigh crease.

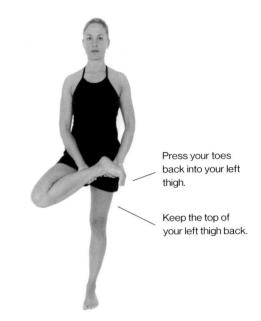

Press your toes back into your left thigh.

Keep the top of your left thigh back.

Keep your right foot drawn in close in the thigh crease.

4 Bend forward at the waist and touch the floor.

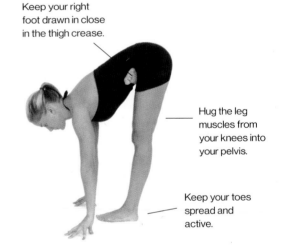

Hug the leg muscles from your knees into your pelvis.

Keep your toes spread and active.

5 Keeping your hands in contact with the floor, bend your left knee and sit down on your left heel. Place your left heel near the perineum, up off the floor.

6 Balance on your left heel by bringing your hands up to prayer position. Hold for several breaths, then come out of the pose and repeat on the other side.

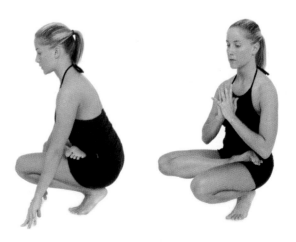

Boat

Navasana

Counterposes
- Knees-to-Chest (Apanasana)

Drishti
- Forward, at big toes

Physical Benefits
- Builds core strength
- Improves balance, digestion, and circulation
- Strengthens the legs, hips, groin, abdomen, and arms
- Lengthens the spine and neck
- Opens the chest, shoulders, and throat
- Improves posture

Mental Benefits
- Improves concentration
- Develops focus

Contraindications
- Pregnancy (keep knees bent)
- Neck or low back pain/ injury (keep knees bent)
- Low blood pressure
- Menstruation

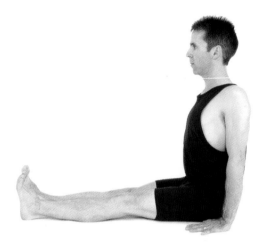

1 Sit in Dandasana (see page 170).

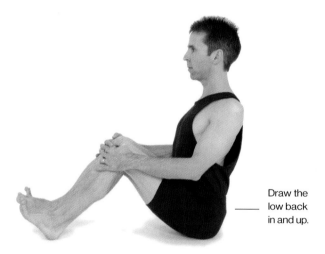

Draw the low back in and up.

2 Bend your knees and place your hands on your upper shins. Inhale and lengthen from the core of your pelvis up through the crown of your head. Draw in muscularly from your hands up to your shoulders and bring your shoulder blades onto your back behind your heart.

3 Maintain all the actions from step 2. Lean your torso back and balance on your buttocks between your sitting bones and your tailbone.

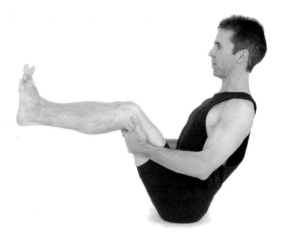

4 Exhale and bring your legs out straight at an upward angle while simultaneously stretching your arms forward. Extend from the core of your pelvis out through the inseam of your legs and up through the top of your head. Draw from your fingers up into your shoulders and bring the shoulder blades even more onto your back.

Flex your feet, spread your toes, and press through the ball of the big toe.

Keep your arms parallel to the floor with the palms facing inward.

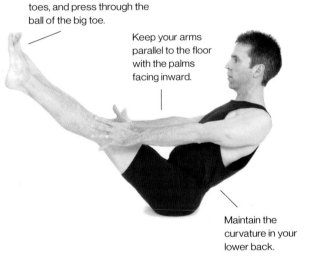

5 Hold for 30 to 60 seconds, or as long as you can without losing the form of the pose, then release.

Maintain the curvature in your lower back.

Gentle Variation

Follow steps 1 through 5 but place a strap just below your toes. Press the balls of your feet into the strap creating resistance by pulling the ends of the strap with your hands.

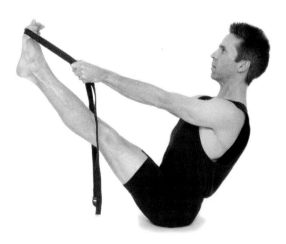

Revolved Half-Moon

Parivrtta Ardha Chandrasana

Counterpose
- Standing Forward Bend (Uttanasana)

Drishti
- Upward
- Forward
- At the floor

Physical Benefits
- Tones the abdominal muscles
- Strengthens the feet, ankles, knees, and thighs
- Stretches the hamstrings
- Opens the chest and lungs
- Stimulates digestion and circulation
- Improves balance

Mental Benefits
- Builds focus
- Develops willpower
- Stimulates the mind

Contraindications
- Knee injury
- Neck injury (keep gaze to the floor)
- Low blood pressure
- Headache

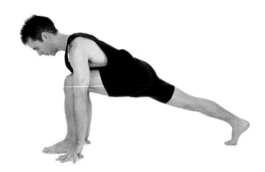

1 Start in a Lunge with your left foot forward and your right leg straight.

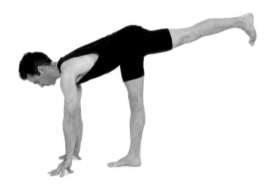

2 Inhale and lift up to balancing on your right leg and the fingertips of both hands.

3 Bring your right hand to your hip. Inhale, shrug your right shoulder to your right ear, and roll it back, twisting to open your chest to the right. Extend your right arm directly above your right shoulder. Exhale and extend from your pelvis out through your feet. Inhale; extend from your low belly up through your head and out through your arms.

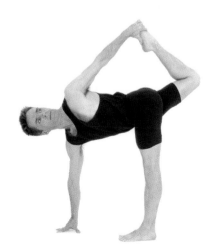

Keep your left leg lifted to hip height.

Keep your left hand directly below your left shoulder.

Engage your leg muscles to the bone and draw the muscles from the floor up to your pelvis.

4 Hold for several breaths, then look down and place both hands on the floor. Exhale and lower your right leg down. Place your hands on your hips, root through your feet into the floor, inhale, and come up to standing. Repeat on the other side.

Gentle Variation

Follow steps 1 through 4. Place a block underneath your bottom hand for support.

Other Variations

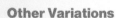

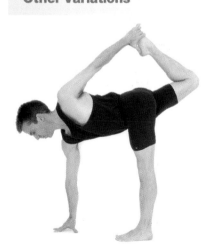

Standing Extended-Leg Stretch

Utthita Hasta Padangusthasana

Counterpose

▶ Mountain (Tadasana)

Drishti

▶ Forward

▶ Up the leg, at the big toe

▶ Over the shoulder of the standing leg

Physical Benefits

▶ Improves balance

▶ Strengthens the arches, ankles, calves, and thighs

▶ Stretches the hamstrings

▶ Lengthens the spine

Mental Benefits

▶ Builds focus

▶ Develops willpower

▶ Stimulates the mind

▶ Cultivates poise

Contraindications

▶ Knee, ankle, or hip injury (keep knee into chest)

▶ Vertigo

▶ Hernia

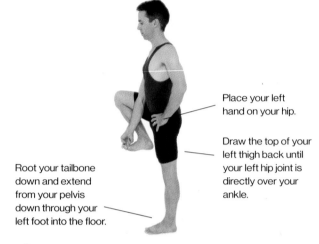

Place your left hand on your hip.

Draw the top of your left thigh back until your left hip joint is directly over your ankle.

Root your tailbone down and extend from your pelvis down through your left foot into the floor.

1 Stand in Tadasana (see page 28). Spread your toes and root down into the floor through all four corners of your feet. Inhale and draw muscularly from your feet up into the core of your pelvis. Bend your right leg, bring your arm to the inside of the leg, and grasp your big toe with the first two fingers of your right hand.

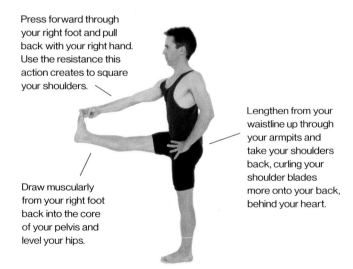

Press forward through your right foot and pull back with your right hand. Use the resistance this action creates to square your shoulders.

Lengthen from your waistline up through your armpits and take your shoulders back, curling your shoulder blades more onto your back, behind your heart.

Draw muscularly from your right foot back into the core of your pelvis and level your hips.

2 Lower your right hip to bring your hip bones level. Maintain steadiness in your legs and torso. Exhale and stretch your right leg straight and parallel with the floor.

3 Externally spiral (rotate) your right leg and descend your right hip. Exhale and take your right leg out to the right.

Root your tailbone down and extend from your low belly up through the crown of your head.

Draw your shoulder blades more onto your back.

Press the ball of your big toe away from your torso against the resistance of your fingers.

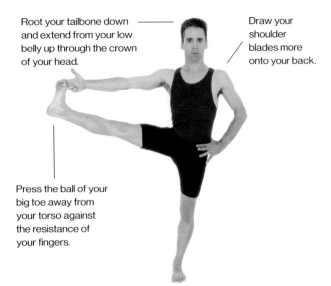

4 Extend your left arm out, parallel with the floor, with your palm facing down. Turn your gaze to the left. Hold for a few breaths. Release and repeat on the other side.

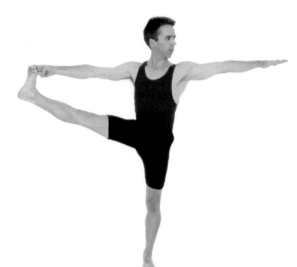

Gentle Variation

Follow steps 1 and 2. Wrap a strap around your left foot, just below the toes.

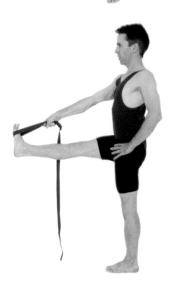

Warrior III

Virabhadrasana III

Counterpose
▶ Standing Forward Bend
(Uttanasana)

Drishti
▶ Straight ahead
▶ At the floor

Physical Benefits
▶ Strengthens the feet,
ankles, calves, knees, and
thighs
▶ Improves circulation
▶ Enhances muscular
endurance
▶ Improves balance
▶ Stretches the hips and groin

Mental Benefits
▶ Builds focus
▶ Develops willpower
▶ Stimulates the mind

Contraindications
▶ Ankle injury
▶ Knee injury

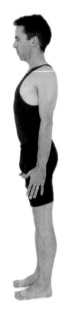

1 Stand in Tadasana (page 28).

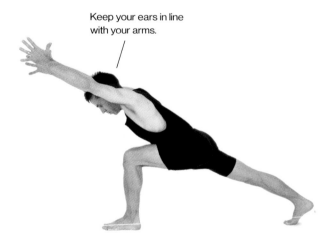

Keep your ears in line
with your arms.

2 Exhale, step your left foot forward, and bend
your knee to 90 degrees. Bend your trunk forward
and bring your belly to your thigh. Extend your
arms alongside your ears.

3 Inhale, lift your torso up buoyantly like a hot air balloon, and balance on your left leg as you extend your right leg back. Rotate your right leg so that your knee and foot point directly toward the floor. Extend from your right groin out through your right inner ankle.

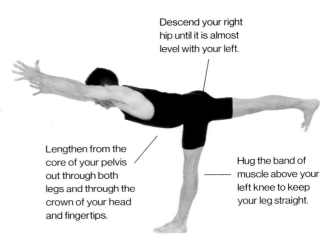

Descend your right hip until it is almost level with your left.

Lengthen from the core of your pelvis out through both legs and through the crown of your head and fingertips.

Hug the band of muscle above your left knee to keep your leg straight.

4 Hold for several breaths. Continue to strongly engage the muscles of the legs to come out of the pose and lower slowly to an extended lunge with your fingertips on the floor by your left ankle. Repeat on the other side.

Dancer

Natarajasana

Counterpose
- Standing Forward Bend (Uttanasana)

Drishti
- Straight ahead, at fingertips

Physical Benefits
- Helps reduce menstrual discomfort
- Develops poise
- Strengthens the leg muscles and arches of feet
- Opens the chest and shoulders
- Increases lung capacity
- Tones the spine

Mental Benefits
- Energizes the mind
- Relieves mild depression and anxiety
- Reduces stress

Contraindications
- Knee injury
- Vertigo
- High blood pressure

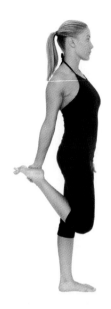

1 Stand in Tadasana (see page 28). Bend your right leg and hold the inside of your foot.

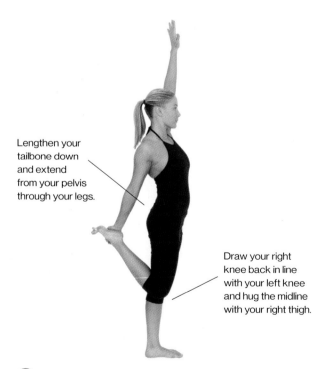

Lengthen your tailbone down and extend from your pelvis through your legs.

Draw your right knee back in line with your left knee and hug the midline with your right thigh.

2 Inhale and extend your left arm up.

3 Exhale and take your right leg back.

Lengthen up through the right side of your body and take your right shoulder back.

Bend forward at your hip joint keeping length in the spine and hips level.

Continue to hug the midline and press your foot into your hand.

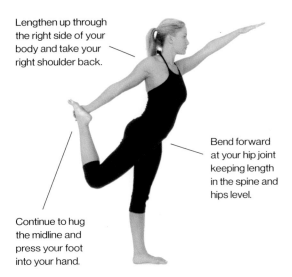

Inhale and extend from the core of your pelvis up through the crown of your head.

4 Exhale, bend at your hips, bring your torso parallel to the floor, and extend your right leg to the sky.

5 Hold for a few breaths, then exhale. Release and repeat on the other side.

Lengthen your tailbone down and extend from the core of your pelvis out through your right leg and down through your left leg.

Hug your leg muscles to the bone, especially engaging the muscles above your right knee.

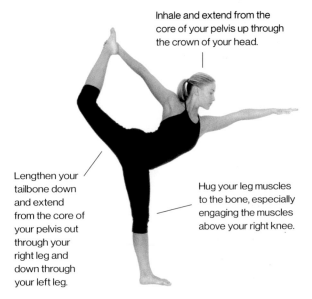

Gentle Variation
Use a strap to hold your foot.

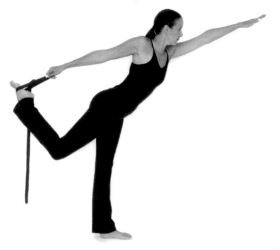

Half-Moon

Ardha Chandrasana

Counterpose
- ▶ Standing Forward Bend (Uttanasana)

Drishti
- ▶ Over the fingertips
- ▶ Forward
- ▶ On floor

Physical Benefits
- ▶ Improves circulation
- ▶ Increases energy to the spine and low back
- ▶ Strengthens the arches, ankles, knees, and thighs
- ▶ Stretches the hamstrings
- ▶ Opens the chest and hips
- ▶ Relieves menstrual discomfort and sciatica
- ▶ Improves balance and coordination

Mental Benefits
- ▶ Builds focus
- ▶ Develops willpower
- ▶ Stimulates the mind
- ▶ Relieves stress

Contraindications
- ▶ Knee injury
- ▶ Neck injury (keep gaze forward or to the floor)
- ▶ Low blood pressure
- ▶ Vertigo

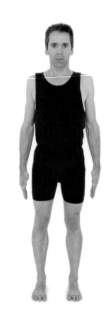

1 Stand in Tadasana (see page 28).

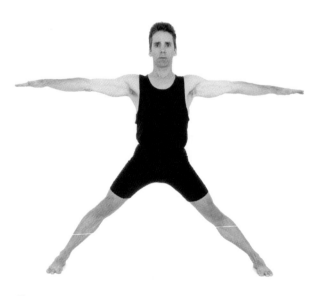

2 Step your feet wide apart. Inhale and extend your arms out to the side.

3 Turn your left foot in slightly; turn your right leg out directly to the side.

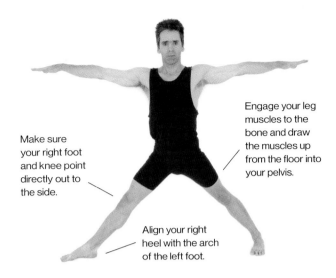

Make sure your right foot and knee point directly out to the side.

Engage your leg muscles to the bone and draw the muscles up from the floor into your pelvis.

Align your right heel with the arch of the left foot.

4 Exhale and bend your right knee and place your right fingertips about 10 to 12 inches in front of your right foot.

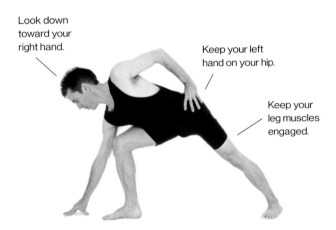

Look down toward your right hand.

Keep your left hand on your hip.

Keep your leg muscles engaged.

5 Inhale and lift so you are balancing on your right leg and hand. Extend your left arm fully above your left shoulder.

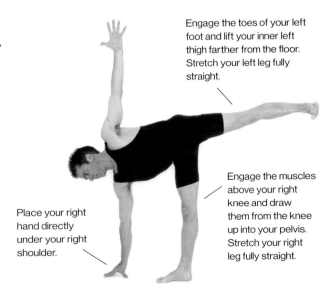

Engage the toes of your left foot and lift your inner left thigh farther from the floor. Stretch your left leg fully straight.

Place your right hand directly under your right shoulder.

Engage the muscles above your right knee and draw them from the knee up into your pelvis. Stretch your right leg fully straight.

6 Keeping your attention to your balance focused in your pelvis, turn your head to look up at your left hand.

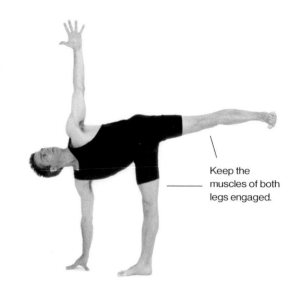

Keep the muscles of both legs engaged.

7 Hold for a few breaths, then bring your left hand to your hip and turn your gaze down to the floor. Exhale, bend your right knee, and slowly bring your left leg down to the floor behind you. Bring your hands to your hips, keep your legs engaged, and slowly come back to Tadasana. Repeat on the other side.

Gentle Variation

Follow steps 1 through 5. Place a block under your lower hand for support in step 4 and keep your top hand on your hip.

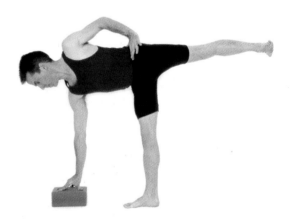

chapter 4

Arm-Balancing Postures

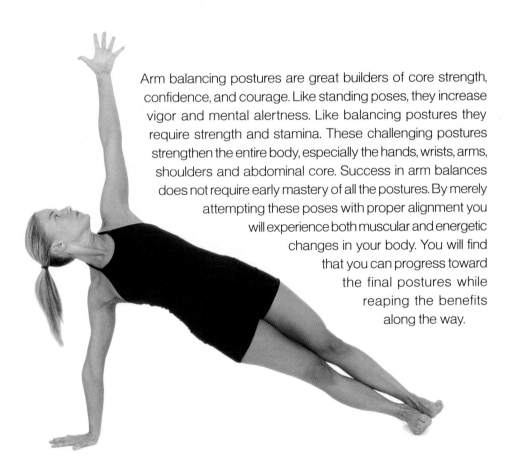

Arm balancing postures are great builders of core strength, confidence, and courage. Like standing poses, they increase vigor and mental alertness. Like balancing postures they require strength and stamina. These challenging postures strengthen the entire body, especially the hands, wrists, arms, shoulders and abdominal core. Success in arm balances does not require early mastery of all the postures. By merely attempting these poses with proper alignment you will experience both muscular and energetic changes in your body. You will find that you can progress toward the final postures while reaping the benefits along the way.

Inclined Plane

Purvottanasana

Counterpose
▶ Seated Forward Bend
(Paschimottanasana)

Drishti
▶ Upward

Physical Benefits
▶ Improves balance
▶ Energizes the body
▶ Opens the chest, shoulders, and throat
▶ Stretches the wrist, shoulder, and ankle joints
▶ Stretches the arm, leg, and back muscles
▶ Increases flexibility and improves posture
▶ Relieves fatigue

Mental Benefits
▶ Improves concentration
▶ Develops focus

Contraindications
▶ Carpal tunnel syndrome
▶ High blood pressure
▶ Wrist, elbow, or shoulder injury
▶ Tendonitis

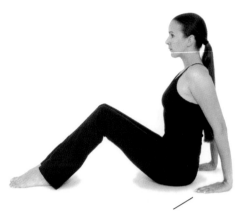

Fingers pointing forward.

1 Sit with your legs straight out in front of you. Bend your knees and place your feet flat on the floor, hip-width apart. Place your hands on the floor behind your hips. Bend your elbows, inhale, and lengthen the side body from your hips up through your armpits. Exhale and draw your shoulder blades onto your back, creating a gentle arch in the back, and straighten your arms.

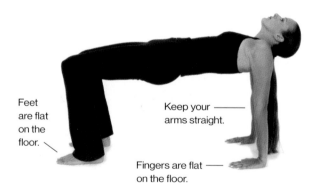

Feet are flat on the floor.

Keep your arms straight.

Fingers are flat on the floor.

2 Inhale, press your hands and feet down, and lift your hips up off the floor. Lengthen your tailbone and extend from the core of your pelvis out through your knees.

3 Fully extend your right leg followed by your left leg. Press the soles of your feet down and draw muscularly from your feet up into your pelvis, keeping your hips lifted.

Keep your legs straight.

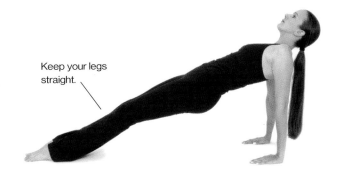

4 Exhale and lengthen from the core of your pelvis out through the crown of your head. Take the sides of your throat back, and curl your head back. Hold this pose for a few breaths. Exhale, bend your knees and arms, and lower your hips to the floor.

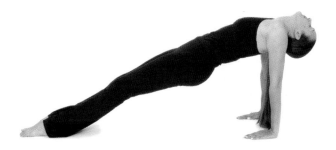

Gentle Variation

Follow the instructions for step 2; lift your hips only as high as you are able.

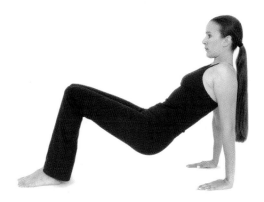

Lateral Inclined Plane

Vasisthasana

Counterpose
- Child's Pose (Balasana)

Drishti
- Up toward raised hand
- Forward
- Down at bottom hand

Physical Benefits
- Improves balance
- Builds core strength
- Strengthens the legs, arms, shoulders, and wrists
- Stretches the wrists
- Lengthens the spine

Mental Benefits
- Improves concentration
- Develops focus

Contraindications
- Wrist, elbow, or shoulder injury
- Carpal tunnel syndrome
- Tendonitis

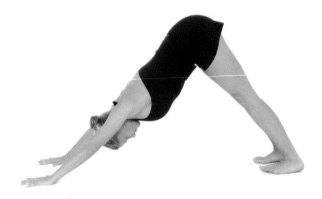

1 Start in Downward-Facing Dog (see page 30).

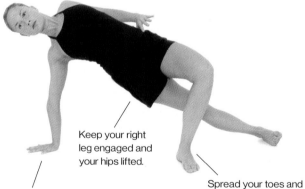

Keep your right leg engaged and your hips lifted.

Spread your toes and keep your ankle square (the foot is at a right angle to your leg and the inner and outer ankle are the same length).

Keeping your right arm at a right angle to your torso, spread your fingers, press your knuckles down, and draw up from back of your right wrist to your shoulder.

2 Bring your right hand to the left along the midline of your body and creating a right angle with your torso. Balance on the outer edge of your right foot. Bend your left knee and place your left foot on the floor in front of your right leg.

3 Stack your left foot on top of your right foot and extend your left arm up.

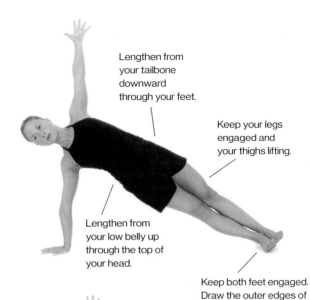

Lengthen from your tailbone downward through your feet.

Keep your legs engaged and your thighs lifting.

Lengthen from your low belly up through the top of your head.

Keep both feet engaged. Draw the outer edges of your feet back toward your knees.

4 Turn to look up toward the fingers of your left hand. Remain in the pose for a few breaths. Exhale and bring your arm down and transition through Downward-Facing Dog repeating the pose on other side.

Gentle Variation

Perform only steps 1 and 2 and hold the pose for a few breaths. Transition to Downward-Facing Dog and repeat the pose on the other side.

Other Variation

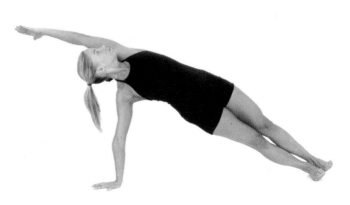

Crane

Bakasana

Counterpose
- Child's Pose (Balasana)

Drishti
- Down and forward toward fingertips

Physical Benefits
- Improves balance and coordination
- Improves digestion
- Strengthens the abdominal muscles, building core strength
- Opens the hips and back
- Strengthens the arms and wrists
- Stretches the wrists

Mental Benefits
- Improves concentration
- Develops focus

Contraindications
- Carpal tunnel syndrome
- Pregnancy
- Wrist or shoulder injury

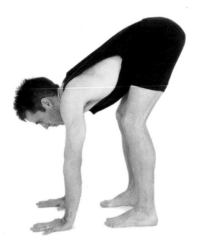

1 Stand with your feet hip-width apart, bend your knees and place your hands flat on the floor.

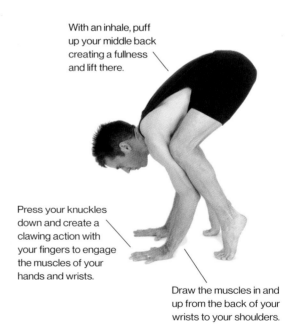

With an inhale, puff up your middle back creating a fullness and lift there.

Press your knuckles down and create a clawing action with your fingers to engage the muscles of your hands and wrists.

Draw the muscles in and up from the back of your wrists to your shoulders.

2 Bend your elbows, bring your knees to the back of your upper arms, come onto your toes, and begin to transfer more weight onto your hands.

3 Lift one leg at a time.

4 Press the inner edges of your feet together, along the big toe side, squeezing your legs to the midline—through the core of the body in line with the spine and between the legs.

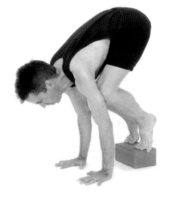

Keep lifting upward into your middle back with the breath.

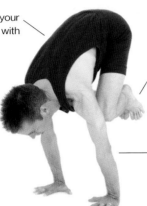

Squeeze the inner edges of your feet and inner thighs together toward the midline.

Straighten your arms.

Gentle Variation

Follow steps 1 through 4 except place your feet on a block to help create more lift in your middle back and hips.

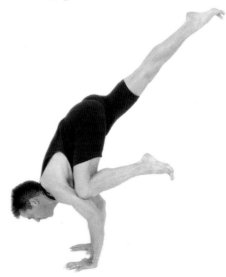

Other Variations

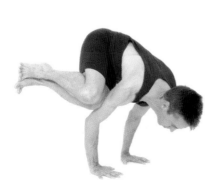

Peacock

Mayurasana

Counterpose
▶ Child's Pose (Balasana)

Drishti
▶ Tip of nose

Physical Benefits
▶ Strengthens the wrists, forearms, and elbows
▶ Lengthens the spine
▶ Tones the abdominal muscles
▶ Stimulates digestion
▶ Improves circulation to the intestines, colon, stomach, spleen, kidneys, and liver
▶ Cultivates balance and poise

Mental Benefits
▶ Improves concentration
▶ Develops focus

Contraindications
▶ Low or high blood pressure
▶ Insomnia
▶ Migraine
▶ Carpal tunnel syndrome

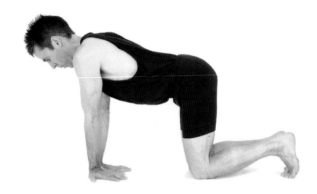

1 Start on your hands and knees with your fingers facing back toward your knees and your little fingers touching.

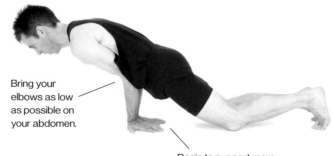

Bring your elbows as low as possible on your abdomen.

Begin to support more body weight on your hands.

2 Bend your elbows, keep your hands together, and lean forward to rest your abdomen on your elbows and your chest on your upper arms. Women may have to separate their upper arms more to leave space and not compress the breasts.

3 Straighten your legs and bring your weight forward to balance on your arms and hands.

Spread your toes to help engage the legs and create lift.

Keep the muscles of the torso fully engaged.

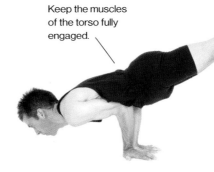

Engage your legs fully, lifting from your inner thighs.

Gentle Variation

Keep your knees and feet touching the floor and practice brief lifts of your torso.

Other Variation

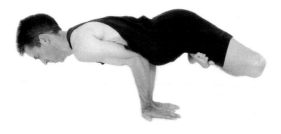

Four-Limbed Staff

Chaturanga Dandasana

Counterpose

▶ Downward-Facing Dog
(Adho Mukha Svanasana)

Drishti

▶ On the floor

▶ Forward

Physical Benefits

▶ Strengthens the legs,
buttocks, back, abdominals,
shoulders, arms, and wrists

▶ Improves circulation and
digestion

▶ Helps relieve minor
tendonitis and fatigue

▶ Energizes the body

▶ Builds core strength

Mental Benefits

▶ Improves concentration

▶ Develops focus

Contraindications

▶ Carpal tunnel syndrome

▶ Pregnancy (use the gentle
variation)

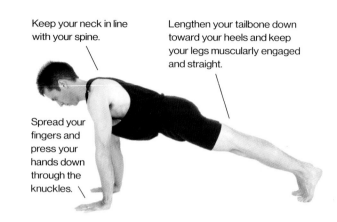

Keep your neck in line with your spine.

Lengthen your tailbone down toward your heels and keep your legs muscularly engaged and straight.

Spread your fingers and press your hands down through the knuckles.

1 Bring your body into a plank pose. Place your hands under your shoulders with your arms straight. Extend your legs back and flex your feet. Lift the sides of your waistline up. Maintaining the lift, draw your shoulder blades onto your back.

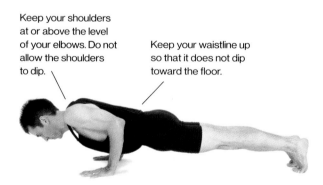

Keep your shoulders at or above the level of your elbows. Do not allow the shoulders to dip.

Keep your waistline up so that it does not dip toward the floor.

2 Maintain all of the actions from step 1. Exhale and lower your body until your upper arms are parallel with the floor.

3 Hold for a few breaths. Release by lowering your body to the floor.

Gentle Variation

Follow steps 1 and 2, but keep your knees on the floor.

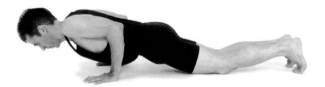

chapter 5

Inverted Postures

Inverted poses reverse the effects of gravity, revitalizing the entire system. They replenish the brain and stimulate the organs and glandular system by reversing the normal flow of blood and lymph. After an inversion the normal circulatory patterns are restored with a new vitality. Inversions also strengthen the upper body and nervous system and improve digestion and elimination. They require focus and concentration and create clarity of perception, equipoise, and calm. They are usually not practiced during pregnancy and are not to be practiced during menstruation.

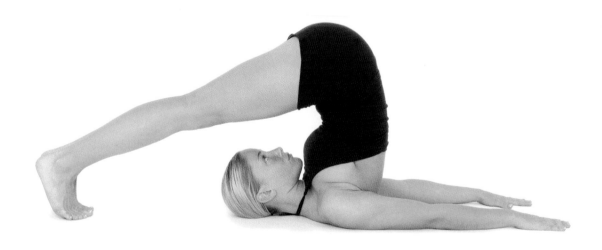

Shoulder Stand

Sarvangasana

Counterpose
▷ Rest on your back

Drishti
▷ At the toes

Physical Benefits
▷ Stretches and strengthens the neck, shoulders, and rhomboids
▷ Alleviates insomnia
▷ Relieves sinus pressure
▷ Improves circulation
▷ Helps relieve menopausal discomfort
▷ Stimulates thyroid, parathyroid, and prostate function
▷ Reduces varicose veins

Mental Benefits
▷ Relieves mild depression and stress
▷ Calms the mind

Contraindications
▷ Neck or disk injury (use the gentle variation)
▷ Menstruation
▷ First trimester of pregnancy
▷ High blood pressure

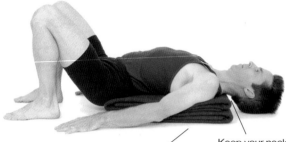

Fold the blankets such that they give a firm surface with crisp edges.

Keep your neck and head off the blanket to maintain the natural curve in your cervical spine.

1 Lie on your back, placing the tops of your shoulders on the edge of two or three folded blankets. Bend your knees and place your feet flat on the floor.

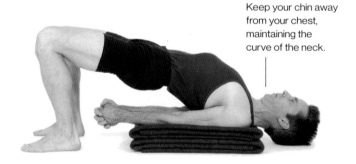

Keep your chin away from your chest, maintaining the curve of the neck.

2 Lift your hips off the blanket and clasp your hands underneath your body. Walk your shoulders one at a time more toward your spine and closer to your ears. This creates lift under your neck and shoulder blades.

3 Lower your hips to the blanket. Bring your legs over your head and touch your feet to the floor in Halasana (Plow) pose (see page 92).

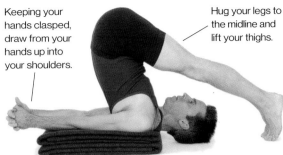

Keeping your hands clasped, draw from your hands up into your shoulders.

Hug your legs to the midline and lift your thighs.

4 Bring your hands onto your back and lift your legs upward. Rotate your upper thighs inward and take your thighs back. Keeping your thighs back, lengthen your tailbone toward your feet.

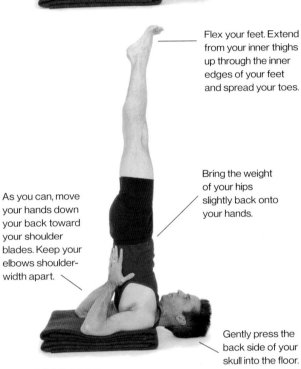

Flex your feet. Extend from your inner thighs up through the inner edges of your feet and spread your toes.

As you can, move your hands down your back toward your shoulder blades. Keep your elbows shoulder-width apart.

Bring the weight of your hips slightly back onto your hands.

Gently press the back side of your skull into the floor.

Gentle Variation

Perform Legs-Up-the-Wall (see page 94); lie with your legs up the wall and your hips on a bolster or blanket.

Other Variations

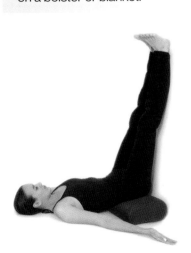

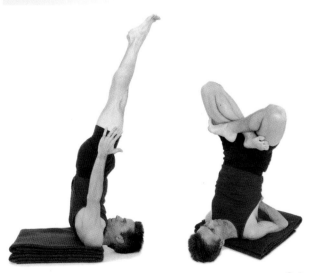

Plow

Halasana

Counterpose

▷ Rest on your back

Drishti

▷ At the top of thighs

Physical Benefits

▷ Assists in relieving backache

▷ Stimulates the thyroid and parathyroid glands

▷ Stretches the shoulders

▷ Strengthens the spine

▷ Alleviates insomnia

▷ Helps relieve menopausal discomfort

Mental Benefits

▷ Calms the mind

▷ Reduces mild stress and anxiety

Contraindications

▷ Menstruation

▷ Neck injury (use the gentle variation)

▷ Asthma

▷ Pregnancy

▷ High blood pressure

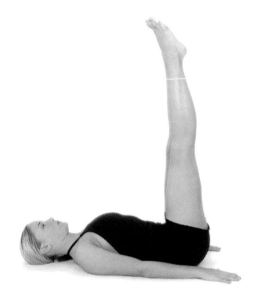

1 Lying flat on the floor, extend your legs vertically by bending your knees toward your chest and then extending your feet toward the ceiling.

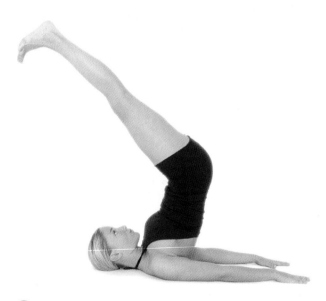

2 Inhale deeply, press your hands into the floor, and swing your legs forward over your head.

3 Bring your toes to the floor and keep your hips above your shoulders. Stay in the pose for several breaths. Using your hands for support, slowly roll onto your back and come out of the pose.

Spread your toes, hug your legs to the midline (through the core of the body in line with the spine), and lift your thighs toward the ceiling.

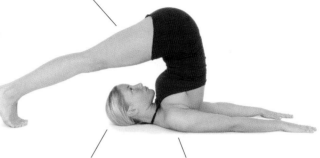

Press the back of your head into the floor and take your chin away from your chest to increase the curve in your neck.

Draw in muscularly from your hands to your shoulders, bringing your shoulder blades strongly onto your back.

Gentle Variation

Follow steps 1 through 3 except place two folded blankets under your shoulders. Keep your head and neck on the floor and maintain the natural curve in the neck.

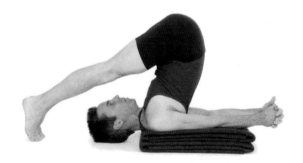

Other Variations

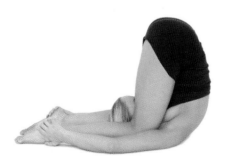

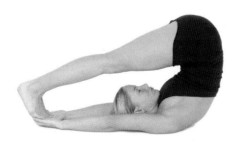

Legs-Up-the-Wall

Viparita Karani

Counterpose
▷ Corpse (Savasana)

Drishti
▷ Eyes closed

Physical Benefits
▷ Relieves fatigue in the legs and feet
▷ Prevents edema and varicose veins
▷ Soothes the nervous system
▷ Relieves mild backache, headache, and insomnia
▷ Relieves symptoms of arthritis
▷ Alleviates urinary and respiratory disorders
▷ Increases circulation

Mental Benefits
▷ Calms the mind
▷ Relieves mild depression, stress, and anxiety

Contraindications
▷ Glaucoma
▷ Serious neck or back injury

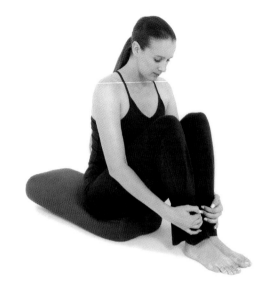

1 Sit on a bolster or folded blankets with your left hip against the wall. Bend your knees.

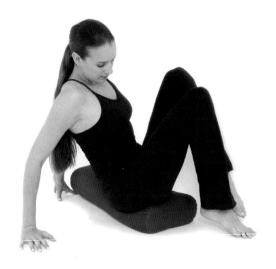

2 Reach your hands behind your body and lean your torso backward.

3 Lean back and rest on your hands as you swivel your hips and bring your feet up the wall.

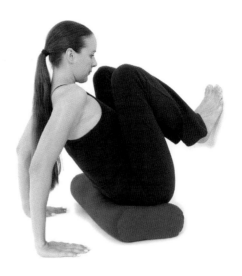

4 Keep your buttocks close to the wall and lie down on your back. Rest with your arms out to the sides, palms up. Close your eyes and relax in the pose, breathing softly and evenly.

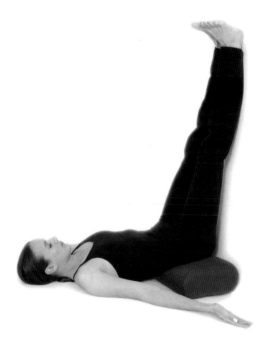

Head Stand

Sirsasana

Counterpose

▶ Child's Pose (Balasana)

Drishti

▶ Tip of nose

Physical Benefits

▶ Stimulates the prostate and pituitary glands

▶ Improves digestion

▶ Strengthens the spinal muscles

▶ Strengthens the arms, legs, and abdomen

▶ Improves circulation

▶ Reduces varicose veins

Mental Benefits

▶ Calms the mind

▶ Relieves mild stress and anxiety

Contraindications

▶ Heart conditions

▶ Neck or back injury

▶ Menstruation

▶ High blood pressure

▶ Headache

▶ Pregnancy (during the first trimester)

▶ Glaucoma

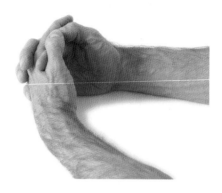

1 Start on your knees with your forearms on the floor. Tightly interlace your fingers, placing special emphasis on the index and middle fingers. Form a cup shape with your hands. Firmly press the pinky sides of your hands on the floor and anchor your forearms down. Keep your wrists perpendicular to the floor.

The back of your head touches your hands at the heel of the hands.

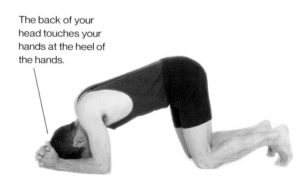

2 Walk your knees a few inches behind your hips and lengthen the sides of your body from your waistline up through your shoulders. Exhale, melt your heart toward the floor and engage your shoulder blades on your back. Place the crown of your head on the floor.

3 Straighten your legs and walk your feet in toward your head. Position your hips directly over your shoulders while keeping your shoulder blades engaged on your back.

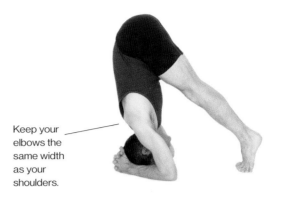

Keep your elbows the same width as your shoulders.

4 Bend your knees and use the strength of your abdominal core to gently lift or hop your feet off the floor.

5 Hug your legs together; lift your knees directly over your shoulders and lengthen your tailbone up toward the ceiling. Distribute the weight between your head and your forearms. Actively extend your head into the floor to avoid compressing your neck.

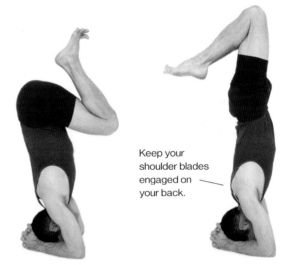

Keep your shoulder blades engaged on your back.

6 Extend your legs straight up over your torso. Hug your thighs to the midline and straighten your legs. Flex your feet, spread your toes, and draw the little-toe sides of your feet toward the floor.

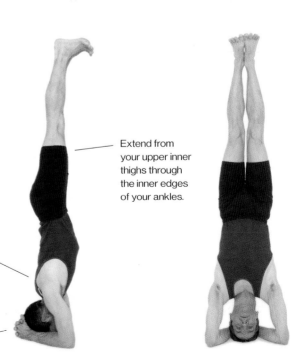

Extend from your upper inner thighs through the inner edges of your ankles.

Press your forearms down while drawing your shoulder blades onto your back and up, toward your feet.

Extend from your palate down through the crown of your head.

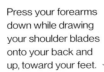

Gentle Variation

As a strengthener to prepare for the Head Stand, perform steps 1 and 2 except keep your head off the floor, your hips behind your shoulders at an angle, and engage your shoulder blades strongly on your back.

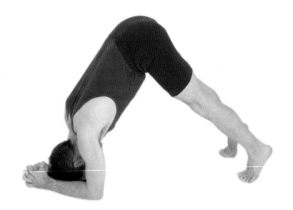

Other Variations

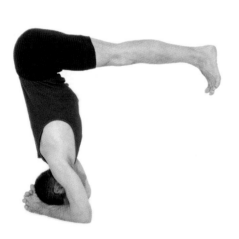

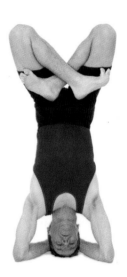

chapter 6

Backward-Bending Postures

Backbends are rejuvenating, strengthening, and awakening. They are most effective at opening the upper back, chest, shoulders, and front groin, and increasing spinal flexibility. Backbends release held emotional energy better than any other class of asanas. They keep the spine supple while developing strength in the back, legs, and shoulders. Backbends should not be practiced close to the time for sleep as they are heating and invigorating. They should be followed by a series of cooling poses such as twists or forward bends to allow the spine to realign.

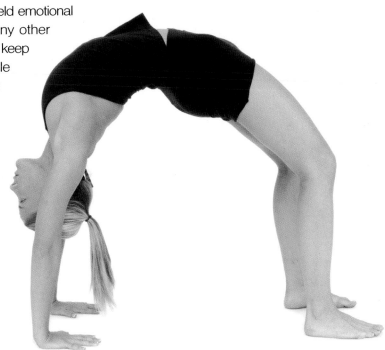

Cobra

Bhujangasana

Counterposes
- Child's Pose (Balasana)
- Lying on belly

Drishti
- Forward
- Upward

Physical Benefits
- Improves posture
- Stimulates the circulatory, digestive, and lymphatic systems
- Opens the chest, shoulders, and throat
- Lengthens the spine and increases spinal flexibility
- Strengthens the low back, shoulders, and legs
- Reduces fatigue

Mental Benefits
- Energizes the mind
- Relieves mild depression and anxiety
- Reduces stress

Contraindications
- Pregnancy
- High blood pressure
- Severe spinal or neck injury

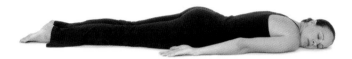

1 Lie on your belly.

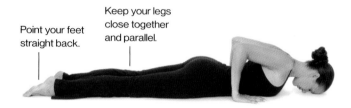

Point your feet straight back.

Keep your legs close together and parallel.

2 Bring your forehead to the floor. Bend your elbows, place your palms near the lower ribs, and keep your lower arms perpendicular to the floor. Exhale, press down with your hands, lengthen through the side body, and lift the head of your arm bones up away from the floor. Draw your shoulder blades onto your back.

From the core of your pelvis, extend up the spine through the crown of your head.

Draw the bottom tips of your shoulder blades into your back and lift your chest from behind your heart.

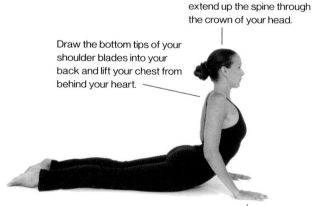

Press your knuckles down and drag back with your hands against the resistance of the floor.

3 Press all ten toenails down and draw muscularly from your feet up into the core of your pelvis. Anchor your tailbone down. On your next inhalation, press your hands down and lengthen from the waistline up into the armpits. Lift your torso up and pin the heads of your arm bones back.

4 Keeping your neck long, slide the sides of your throat back and curl your neck to look up.

5 Hold for a few breaths. Exhale, release, and rest on your belly.

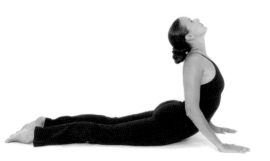

Gentle Variation

Follow steps 1 through 3. Keep your forearms on the floor.

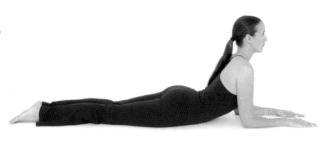

Upward-Facing Dog

Urdhva Mukha Svanasana

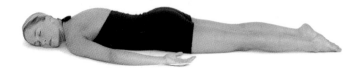

Counterposes
- ▶ Downward-Facing Dog (Adho Mukha Svanasana)
- ▶ Child's Pose (Balasana)

Drishti
- ▶ Forward
- ▶ Upward

Physical Benefits
- ▶ Strengthens the legs, buttocks, torso, shoulders, arms, and wrists
- ▶ Opens the chest, increasing lung capacity
- ▶ Stretches the shoulders and back
- ▶ Lengthens the spine and opens the abdominal cavity
- ▶ Stimulates the digestive and lymphatic systems
- ▶ Improves posture

Mental Benefits
- ▶ Energizes the mind
- ▶ Relieves mild depression and anxiety
- ▶ Creates focus

Contraindications
- ▶ Back or neck injury (use the gentle variation)
- ▶ Pregnancy (after the first trimester)
- ▶ Carpal tunnel syndrome

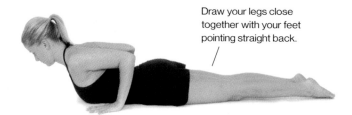

1 Lie on your belly.

Draw your legs close together with your feet pointing straight back.

2 Bend your arms and slide your palms back until your lower arms are perpendicular to the floor. Inhale and lengthen the sides of your body shrugging your shoulders up towards your ears. Lift your shoulders up away from the floor and bring your shoulder blades more onto your back behind your heart.

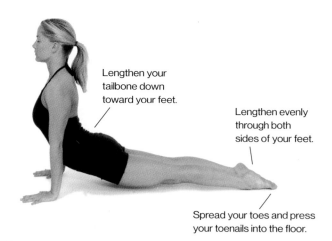

Lengthen your tailbone down toward your feet.

Lengthen evenly through both sides of your feet.

Spread your toes and press your toenails into the floor.

3 Exhale, press your hands down, lengthen up through the sides of your body, and draw the head of your arm bones backward. Draw your shoulder blades securely onto your back and straighten your arms. Engage the muscles above your knees and lift your legs off the floor.

4 Press your knuckles into the floor and pull your hands back toward your feet against the resistance of the floor. Slide your body and legs forward slightly between your hands. Lengthen the sides of your body from your waistline up to your armpits and take the head of your arm bones back even more. Keeping your neck long, slide the sides of your throat back and curl your neck to look up. Remain in the pose for a few breaths, then slowly release back down to the floor.

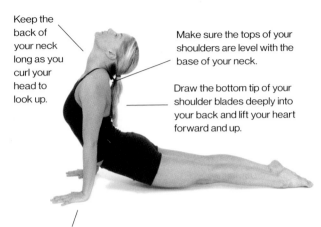

Keep the back of your neck long as you curl your head to look up.

Make sure the tops of your shoulders are level with the base of your neck.

Draw the bottom tip of your shoulder blades deeply into your back and lift your heart forward and up.

Actively press your knuckles and fingertips down and engage the muscles of your arms.

Gentle Variation

Follow the preceding instructions, keeping your thighs on the floor.

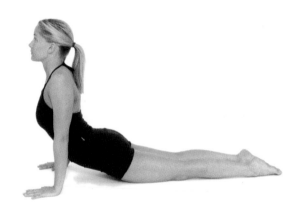

Camel

Ustrasana

Counterposes

▷ Standing Forward Bend (Uttanasana)

▷ Child's Pose (Balasana)

Drishti

▷ Upward

▷ Closed

Physical Benefits

▷ Stretches the thighs, torso, chest, shoulders, and throat

▷ Strengthens the legs, pelvis, and lower back region

▷ Opens the hips and hip flexors

▷ Aids digestion

▷ Stimulates circulation

▷ Increases spinal flexibility

▷ Improves posture

Mental Benefits

▷ Energizes the mind

▷ Relieves mild depression and anxiety

▷ Relieves stress

Contraindications

▷ Spinal or neck injury

▷ Low blood pressure

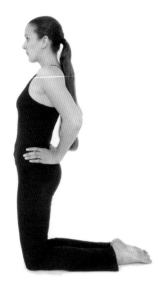

1 Kneel on the floor with your thighs parallel and rest your palms on your hips. Point your feet straight back and press your toenails into the floor. Inhale and take your thighs backward. On the next exhalation, scoop your tailbone to lengthen your lower back.

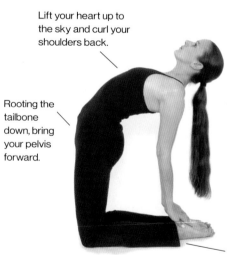

Lift your heart up to the sky and curl your shoulders back.

Rooting the tailbone down, bring your pelvis forward.

Press your shins into the floor.

2 Inhale and extend from your pelvis through your head. Exhale and reach back to place your right hand on your right heel. Repeat with your left hand.

3 Keep your neck elongated and slide the sides of your throat straight back. Maintaining the length in your neck curl your head backwards.

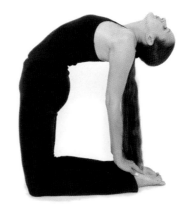

4 Slide your hands down to the soles of your feet. Remain in this position for a few breaths. Exhale, powerfully root down through your shins into the floor, and lift from behind your heart and keep your head back as you come up. Rest by sitting back on your heels for a few breaths.

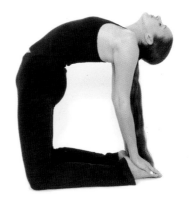

Gentle Variation

Follow steps 1 through 4, but place a block on the outside of each ankle and rest your hands on the blocks instead of on your feet.

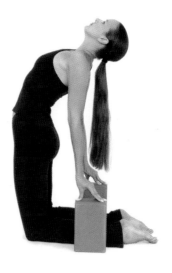

Bridge

Setu Banda Sarvangasana

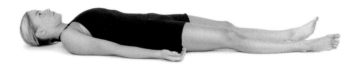

Counterpose
▶ Knees-to-Chest
  (Apanasana)

Drishti
▶ Upward
▶ Closed

Physical Benefits
▶ Improves flexibility in the
  spine and shoulders
▶ Stimulates the nervous
  system
▶ Aids digestion
▶ Opens the chest, neck, and
  shoulders
▶ Stimulates the thyroid and
  parathyroid glands
▶ Increases lung capacity
▶ Relieves menstrual and
  menopausal discomfort
▶ Relieves high blood
  pressure, asthma, and
  sinusitis
▶ Reduces fatigue

Mental Benefits
▶ Energizes the mind
▶ Relieves mild depression
  and anxiety
▶ Reduces stress

Contraindications
▶ Neck or shoulder injury (use
  the gentle variation)
▶ Wrist injury (omit step 4)

1 Lie on your back.

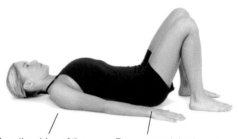

Lengthen the sides of the body, press your shoulders down to the floor, and bring your shoulder blades more onto your back.

Press your sitting bones down into the floor to create a natural curve in the low back.

2 Bend your knees and place your feet parallel to each other and hip-width apart.

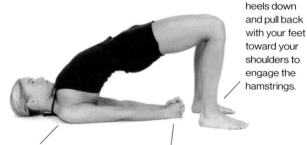

Press your heels down and pull back with your feet toward your shoulders to engage the hamstrings.

Keeping the sides of the your body lengthened, roll both shoulder blades more deeply onto the your back.

Press your hands and arms down to create lift in the hips.

3 Inhale, press your feet into the floor, and lift your hips. Lengthen your tailbone and extend from your pelvis out through your knees. Clasp your hands together under your back and roll your right and left shoulders underneath one at a time, drawing your shoulder blades more onto your back.

4 Press your feet into the floor, inhale, and lift your hips higher. Unclasp your hands, shift your body weight slightly to the right and bring your left hand up to cradle your back ribs with your palm. Repeat this action on the other side. Remain in the pose for a few breaths, then release your hands and slowly lower your hips to the floor.

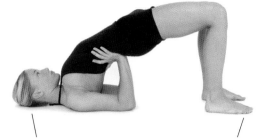

Press the back of your head gently into the floor while lifting your chin away from your chest to create and strengthen the natural curve in the neck.

Spread your toes and press on the inner edges of your feet to draw your thighs parallel.

Gentle Variation

Follow steps 1 through 4. Keep your arms by your sides, palms down. Use a blanket to support your shoulders if needed.

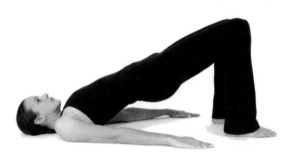

Bow

Counterposes

- Lying on belly
- Child's Pose (Balasana)
- Downward-Facing Dog (Adho Mukha Svanasana)

Drishti

- Forward
- On floor, directly under nose

Physical Benefits

- Stretches the ankles, calves, thighs, and spine
- Strengthens the spine
- Opens the chest and throat
- Aids digestion
- Energizes the body

Mental Benefits

- Energizes the mind
- Relieves mild depression and anxiety
- Reduces stress

Contraindications

- Knee or back injury
- Neck injury (keep your gaze on the floor)
- Pregnancy

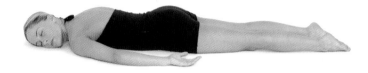

1 Lie on your belly.

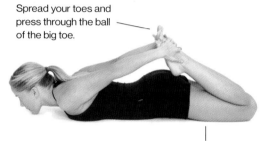

Spread your toes and press through the ball of the big toe.

Keep your thighs parallel.

2 Rest your chin on the floor. Inhale, bend your knees, and hold of the tops of your feet.

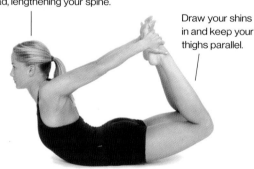

Extend from your pelvis out through the crown of your head, lengthening your spine.

Draw your shins in and keep your thighs parallel.

Only your belly stays on the floor.

3 Inhale, press your knees into the floor, and lift your hips up. Exhale and scoop your tailbone, extending outward toward your knees. Inhale again, and lengthen the sides of your body from your hips to your armpits. Exhale and draw your shoulder blades onto your back behind your heart, press your feet powerfully into your hands, and lift your legs and torso off the floor. Hold the pose for a few breaths. Exhale, lower your knees, release your hands, and rest on your belly.

Gentle Variation

Proceed only through step 1.
Inhale and lift your chest, head,
arms, and legs off the floor.

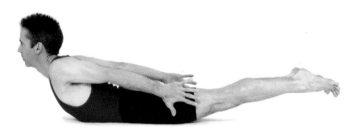

Other Variation

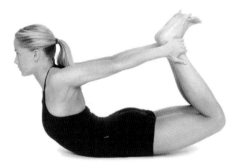

Locust

Salabhasana

Counterposes

- Lying on belly
- Child's Pose (Balasana)

Drishti

- Forward
- Tip of nose

Physical Benefits

- Lengthens the spine
- Opens the chest, shoulders, and throat
- Strengthens the legs, buttocks, shoulders, and arms
- Tones the abdominal cavity and aids digestion
- Stimulates circulation
- Increases flexibility
- Improves posture

Mental Benefits

- Reduces stress
- Relieves mild depression and anxiety
- Energizes the mind

Contraindications

- Headache
- High blood pressure
- Spinal or neck injury (use the gentle variation)
- Pregnancy

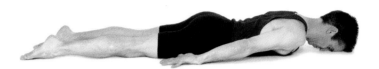

1 Lie on your belly. Stretch your arms straight back by your side. Rest your forehead on the floor.

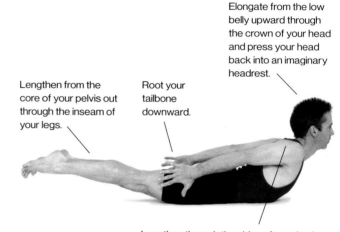

Elongate from the low belly upward through the crown of your head and press your head back into an imaginary headrest.

Lengthen from the core of your pelvis out through the inseam of your legs.

Root your tailbone downward.

Lengthen through the sides of your body and draw your shoulder blades more onto your back behind the your heart.

2 Inhale and simultaneously lift your head, chest, arms, and legs off the floor. Enthusiastically spread your fingers and toes to maintain greater muscle tone. Maintain steady breathing.

3 Remain in the pose for a few breaths and release.

Gentle Variation

Alternately lift one arm and the opposite leg at the same time.

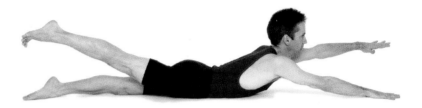

Other Variations

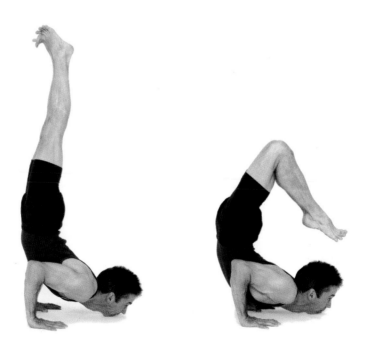

Upward-Facing Bow

Urdva Dhanurasana

Counterposes

▷ Standing Forward Bend (Uttanasana)

▷ Knees-to-Chest (Apanasana)

Drishti

▷ Forward

Physical Benefits

▷ Keeps the spine strong and supple

▷ Stretches the wrists, forearms, shoulders, and spine

▷ Opens the chest

▷ Increases lung capacity

▷ Strengthens the legs, buttocks, back, chest, shoulders, and wrists

▷ Stimulates the lymphatic, digestive, and reproductive systems

▷ Helps relieve infertility, osteoporosis, backache, and asthma

▷ Promotes proper pituitary and thyroid function

▷ Increases stamina

Mental Benefits

▷ Energizes the mind

▷ Relieves mild depression and anxiety

▷ Reduces stress

Contraindications

▷ High or low blood pressure

▷ Carpal tunnel syndrome

▷ Back, neck, or knee injury

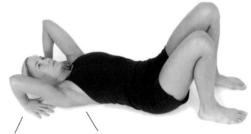

1 Lie on your back.

Press your hands downward and draw muscularly up from the hands to the elbows.

From the elbows, draw the muscles down into your shoulders, hollowing the armpits. Your shoulders will press down into the floor.

2 Bend your knees and place your feet hip-width apart and parallel. Bend your arms and place your palms near your shoulders with the fingers pointing toward the feet.

Press your fingertips into the floor and draw back from your elbows into your shoulders, hollowing the armpits.

Spread your toes and root down evenly through all four corners of your feet. Keep your shins and feet parallel.

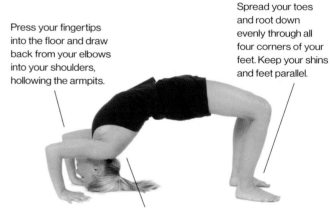

Draw your shoulder blades onto your back, keep your elbows drawing back while you bring your chest forward toward your elbows.

3 Inhale, press your palms into the floor, lift your torso, come to the top of your head, and pause. Widen your hands to at least shoulder-width apart and bring your index fingers parallel. If your shoulders are tight, widen a bit more and slightly spin your fingers outward.

4 Maintain your shoulder integration. Inhale, press your hands and feet into the floor and lift your body up into an arch. Remain in the pose for several breaths. Bend your elbows, bring your chin to your chest and lower onto your shoulders to come out of the pose.

Keep hollowing your armpits back and bring your chest forward.

Press down through the inner edges of your feet and descend your inner groins a couple of inches. Then scoop your tailbone and lengthen it toward your knees.

Make sure your hip bones are level with your bottom ribs.

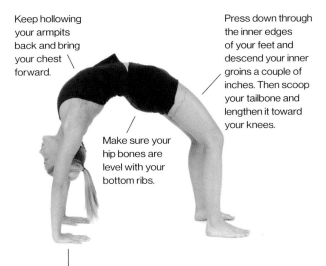

Claw with your fingers and draw up muscularly from your wrists into your shoulders. Straighten your arms.

Gentle Variation

Perform the Bridge (Setu Banda Sarvangasana). See also page 106.

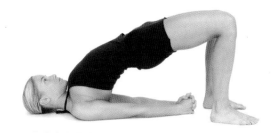

Other Variations

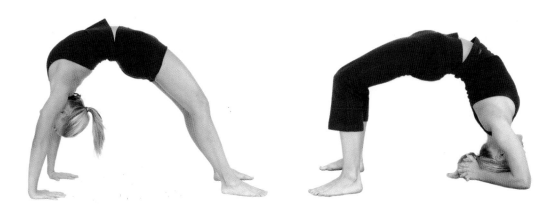

Fish

Matsyasana

Counterpose
▸ Seated Forward Bend
(Paschimottanasana)

Drishti
▸ Upward
▸ Closed

Physical Benefits
▸ Opens the hips, abdominal
cavity, chest, and throat
▸ Stretches the hip flexors
▸ Aids digestion
▸ Helps relieve asthma
▸ Improves posture
▸ Strengthens the muscles of
the upper back, neck, and
shoulders

Mental Benefits
▸ Energizes the mind
▸ Relieves mild depression
and anxiety
▸ Reduces stress

Contraindications
▸ Neck injury
▸ Migraine
▸ High or low blood pressure
▸ Insomnia
▸ Low back injury
▸ Knee or hip injury (use the
gentle variation)

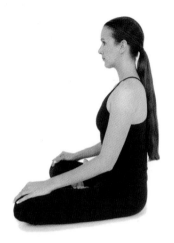

1 Sit with your legs folded in the Lotus pose (see
page 156).

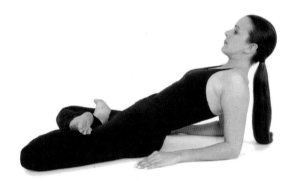

2 Lean your torso back and rest on your elbows.

Lengthen from your
pelvis out through
your knees.

Lift your chest upward.

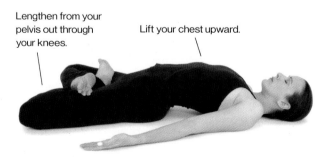

3 Lower your shoulders and the back of your
head to the floor. Bring your arms out straight by
your sides.

4 Inhale, press your elbows down, lift your chest, curl your neck back, and rest the top of your head on the floor. Hold the soles of your feet with your hands. Remain in the pose for several breaths. Come out of the pose by using your elbows for support to lower your back to the floor. Then use your elbows to bring yourself back up to a sitting position and release your legs.

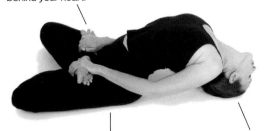

Actively pull your feet and bring your shoulder blades more onto your back behind your heart.

Lengthen your tailbone, stretch the front of your thighs, and extend from your pelvis out through your knees.

Press the back of your head into the floor and back toward your hips, deepening the arch of the back and coming more onto the crown of your head.

Gentle Variation

Follow steps 2 through 4. Keep your legs extended and place your hands against your thighs for support.

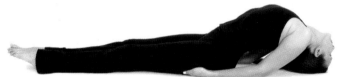

Other Variations

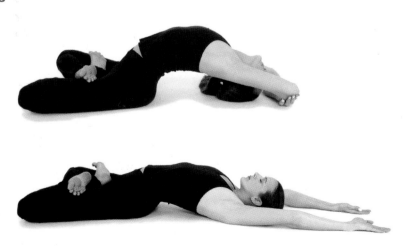

Cat–Cow

Counterpose

▶ Child's Pose (Balasana)

Drishti

▶ At navel
▶ Forward
▶ Upward

Physical Benefits

▶ Increases spinal flexibility
▶ Opens the lower back and abdominal cavity
▶ Aids digestion
▶ Opens the chest, throat, and shoulders
▶ Increases circulation
▶ Stimulates thyroid and parathyroid function
▶ Therapeutic for mild carpal tunnel syndrome, tendonitis, sciatica, and low back injury

Mental Benefits

▶ Energizes the mind
▶ Relieves mild depression and anxiety
▶ Reduces stress

Contraindications

▶ Severe carpal tunnel syndrome

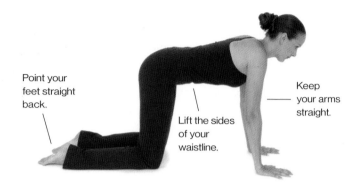

Point your feet straight back.

Lift the sides of your waistline.

Keep your arms straight.

1 Come to all fours with your wrists directly underneath your shoulders and your knees under your hips. Inhale and lengthen from your hips up to your armpits. Spread your fingers and root down through your hands as you draw from the floor up into your shoulders. Bring the shoulder blades onto your back.

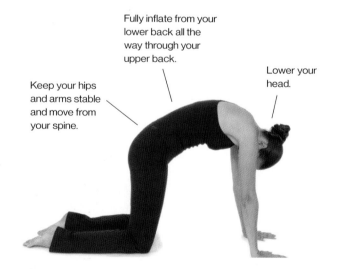

Fully inflate from your lower back all the way through your upper back.

Lower your head.

Keep your hips and arms stable and move from your spine.

2 Exhale, press your hands into the floor, and round your spine up toward the ceiling. Tilt your pelvis down and scoop your tailbone.

3 Inhale and move your spine in the opposite direction, creating concavity in the spine. Tilt your pelvis upward and lift your head.

4 Repeat steps 2 and 3 for five to ten breaths. Push back into Child's Pose and rest for a few breaths.

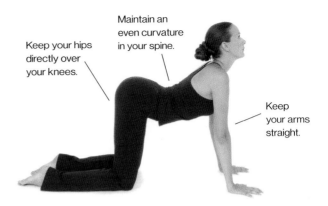

Maintain an even curvature in your spine.

Keep your hips directly over your knees.

Keep your arms straight.

Pigeon

Eka Pada Rajakapotasana

Counterposes
▶ Knees-to-Chest (Apanasana)
▶ Seated Forward Bend (Paschimottanasana)

Drishti
▶ Forward
▶ Upward
▶ Closed

Physical Benefits
▶ Energizes the body
▶ Opens the hip flexors, thighs, chest, and shoulders
▶ Improves circulation to the abdominal cavity and low back
▶ Stimulates the digestive and reproductive systems
▶ Alleviates menstrual and menopausal discomfort
▶ Encourages healthy thyroid, parathyroid, and adrenal function
▶ Therapeutic for low blood pressure, infertility, and headache

Mental Benefits
▶ Energizes the mind
▶ Relieves mild depression and anxiety
▶ Reduces stress

Contraindications
▶ Knee or hip injury
▶ Back or shoulder injury

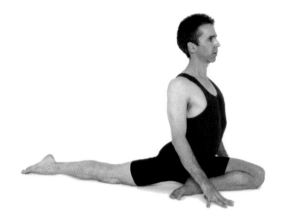

1 Bend your left knee and place your left foot near your right groin with your toes pointed. Extend your right leg straight back, with the front of the thigh, the shin, and the top of the foot resting on the floor. Widen your right hip out to the right and square your hips to the front.

Turn your foot out to the side and grasp across the instep with a strong grip.

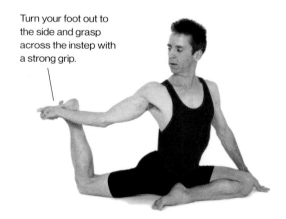

2 Stretch your right arm back with the palm facing up. Inhale and lengthen the sides of your body. Exhale and turn your head, torso, chest, and shoulder to the right. Bend your back leg and grasp your right foot with your right hand.

3 Keep your torso and shoulder turned to the right and draw your right elbow in closer to your side. Inhale and swing your right elbow up. Maintain a strong grip on the foot, swivel the hand, and bring the palm facing down.

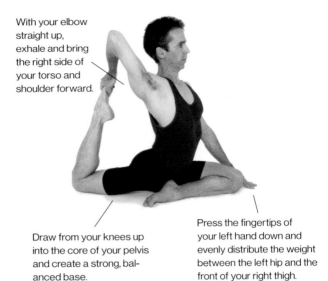

With your elbow straight up, exhale and bring the right side of your torso and shoulder forward.

Draw from your knees up into the core of your pelvis and create a strong, balanced base.

Press the fingertips of your left hand down and evenly distribute the weight between the left hip and the front of your right thigh.

4 Inhale, press your left fingertips into the floor, and lift from your waistline up to your shoulders. Exhale, reach your left arm up and back, and grasp your foot.

Bring your elbows closer together and your upper arms parallel. Powerfully draw from your elbows back into your shoulders, hollowing the armpits.

Press your right foot back into the resistance of your hands to deepen the shoulder stretch.

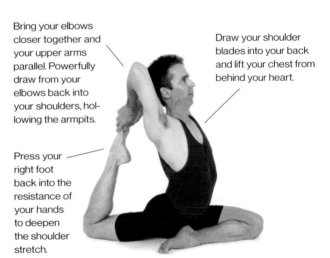

Draw your shoulder blades into your back and lift your chest from behind your heart.

5 Curl your head back to touch your right foot. Remain in the pose for a few breaths, then exhale, release your hands one at a time, and lower your leg. Repeat on the other side.

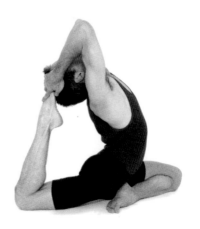

119

Gentle Variation

Follow steps 1 through 4 except use a strap on your foot.

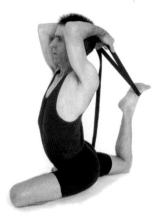

chapter 7

Twisting Postures

Twists are a unique class of postures because they are cooling and soothing after backbends, yet stimulating after forward bends. They are sometimes referred to as "smart poses" because they give the body what it needs to return to homeostasis. Twists massage and tone the entire visceral system and detoxify the glands and organs. In addition, they replenish the circulation to the spinal muscles and disks creating hydration and mobility. They squeeze the abdominal organs as the trunk rotates, allowing fresh blood to surge into organs following a twist. If you are pregnant, be sure to use the gentle versions of the twists.

Gentle Spinal Twist

Drishti
- Forward
- Over shoulder
- Eyes closed

Physical Benefits
- Improves digestion and circulation
- Reduces discomfort from backache, neck pain, and sciatica
- Stretches and strengthens the spine, shoulders, and hips
- Relieves menstrual discomfort
- Stimulates the lymphatic system

Mental Benefits
- Relieves stress, mild depression, and anxiety

Contraindications
- Digestive discomfort
- High or low blood pressure
- Headache

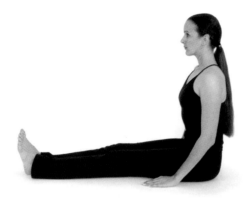

1 Start in Dandasana (see page 170).

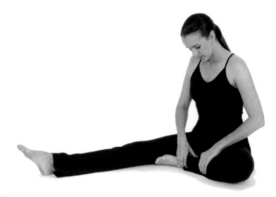

2 Bend your left leg and place your foot in close to the perineum.

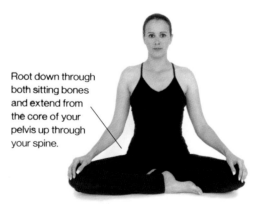

Root down through both sitting bones and extend from the core of your pelvis up through your spine.

3 Bend your right leg, and fold your foot in front of your left ankle, heels in line with each other.

4 Place your left hand on your right knee.

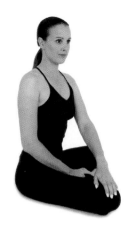

5 Place your right hand behind your back on the floor. Maintain a firm foundation by rooting your sitting bones into the floor. Draw from your knees in toward the core of your pelvis to stabilize the pelvis and sacrum. Inhale and lengthen your spine. Exhale and twist to the right. Hold the pose as long as your breath is steady then return to step 3 and repeat on the other side.

Originate the twist in the core of your pelvis, spiraling the twisting action upward through the spine. The last part of the twist is your head turning to the right.

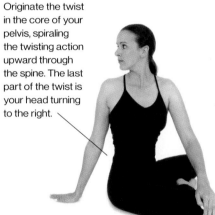

Press your left hand into your right knee for added leverage while twisting.

Gentle Variation

Follow steps 1 through 5, but sit on a folded blanket to elevate your hips. Maintain a straight back by supporting your upper body on your fingertips if necessary.

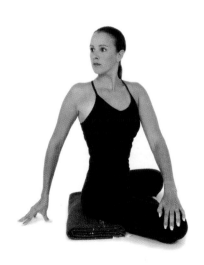

Reclining Spinal Twist

Jathara Parivartanasana

Counterpose
- ▷ Knees-to-Chest (Apanasana)

Drishti
- ▷ Forward
- ▷ Upward

Physical Benefits
- ▷ Stretches the spine and shoulders
- ▷ Improves digestion and circulation
- ▷ Strengthens the lower back
- ▷ Relieves lower backache, neck pain, and sciatica
- ▷ Opens the hips and chest

Mental Benefits
- ▷ Helps relieve stress, mild depression, and anxiety

Contraindications
- ▷ High or low blood pressure
- ▷ Diarrhea
- ▷ Headache
- ▷ Menstruation
- ▷ High blood pressure

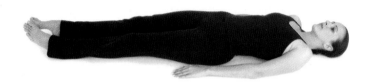

1 Lie on your back with your legs extended.

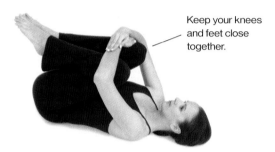

Keep your knees and feet close together.

2 Draw your knees up into your chest and wrap your arms around your legs.

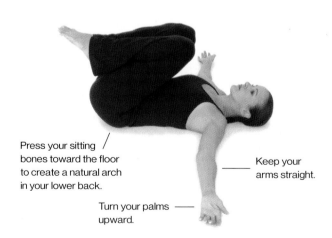

Press your sitting bones toward the floor to create a natural arch in your lower back.

Keep your arms straight.

Turn your palms upward.

3 Keep your knees at your chest and sweep your arms out to the sides.

124

4 Inhale, take your knees to the left, then turn your head to the right.

5 Hold for a few breaths. Inhale, bring your knees and head back to center, and repeat on the other side.

Maintain a natural curve in your lower back.

Extend from the core of your pelvis up through the top of your head.

Press your shoulders back into the floor and draw the shoulder blades onto your back.

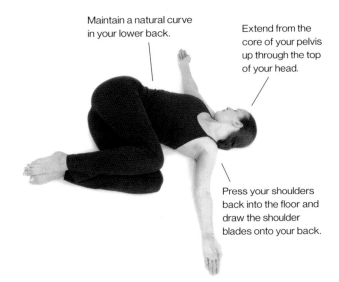

Other Variations

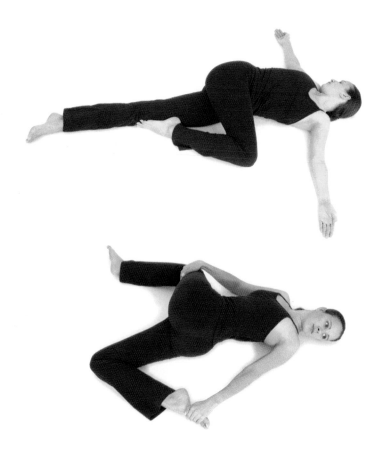

Simple Sitting Twist

Bharadvajasana I

Counterpose
- ▷ Staff (Dandasana)

Drishti
- ▷ Forward
- ▷ Over shoulder
- ▷ Eyes closed

Physical Benefits
- ▷ Opens the chest and neck
- ▷ Stimulates the digestive and lymphatic systems
- ▷ Increases circulation in the spine and abdominal cavity
- ▷ Improves digestion
- ▷ Relieves carpal tunnel syndrome
- ▷ Alleviates sciatica
- ▷ Strengthens the hips, shoulders, and spine
- ▷ Relieves low back and neck discomfort

Mental Benefits
- ▷ Reduces stress
- ▷ Relieves mild anxiety

Contraindications
- ▷ Headache
- ▷ High or low blood pressure
- ▷ Ankle or knee injury (use the gentle variation)

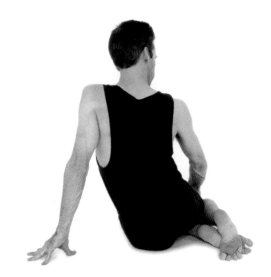

1 Sit on your left hip, bend your knees, and bring both feet to the right of your hips. Point your right foot and place it on the arch of your left foot.

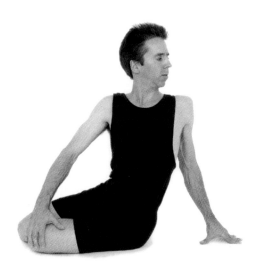

2 Place your right hand on your left knee. Place your left hand behind you and come up onto your fingertips. Inhale and lengthen from the core of your low belly through the top of your head. Keep the length, exhale, and twist to the left.

3 Reach your left arm behind your back and clasp the inside of the right upper arm. Insert your right hand under your left knee, palm facing downward. Inhale and extend from your pelvis up through the crown of your head. Exhale and twist deeply to your left. Turn your head and gaze over your right shoulder.

4 Hold for a few breaths. Release and repeat on the other side.

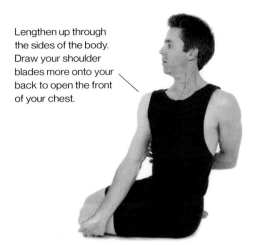

Lengthen up through the sides of the body. Draw your shoulder blades more onto your back to open the front of your chest.

Gentle Variation
Perform Gentle Spinal Twist (see page 122).

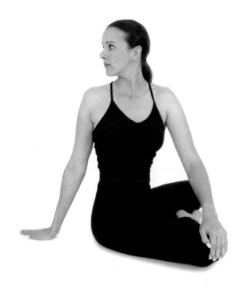

Bound Half-Lotus Twist

Bharadvajasana II

Counterpose
- Staff (Dandasana)

Drishti
- Forward
- Over the shoulder

Physical Benefits
- Strengthens the spine, legs, and arms
- Opens the shoulders and chest
- Tones the abdominal muscles
- Improves digestion and circulation
- Relieves backache and sciatica

Mental Benefits
- Reduces stress
- Relieves anxiety

Contraindications
- Hip, knee, or ankle injury (use the gentle variation)
- Headache
- High or low blood pressure (use the gentle variation)
- Insomnia

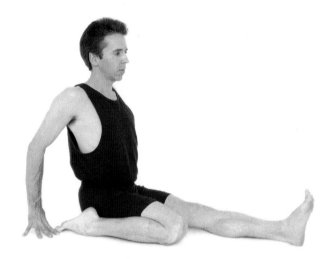

1 Sit on the floor with your legs extended (Dandasana). Fold your right leg back so that your ankle rests outside your hip. Bring your hands back with the fingers facing forward and press your fingers into the floor. Lengthen up through the sides of your body and draw your low back in and up.

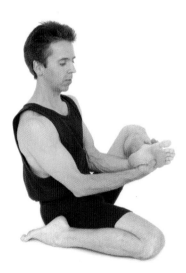

2 Bend your left leg and cradle your ankle and foot in your hands. Keep your left foot flexed and spread your toes.

3 Bring your left leg into half-lotus by drawing your heel in toward your navel. Rest the top of your foot near your right thigh. Bring your right hand behind your back and place your left hand on your right knee.

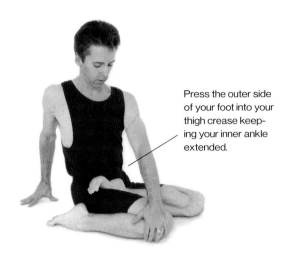

Press the outer side of your foot into your thigh crease keeping your inner ankle extended.

With each inhalation, lengthen your spine.

With each exhalation, deepen the twist.

Actively press your right hand against your knee.

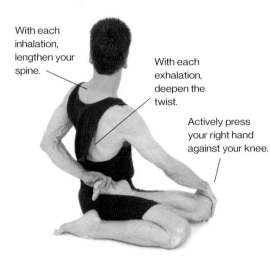

4 Reach around your back and hold your left foot. Place your right hand on your left knee. Inhale, extend from your low belly up through the crown of your head, exhale and twist from your low belly up through your torso.

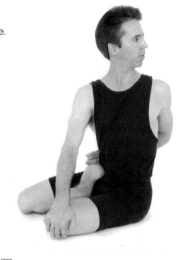

5 Hold for a few breaths. Release and repeat on the other side.

Gentle Variation
Perform Simple Sitting Twist (Bharadvajasana I) on page 126.

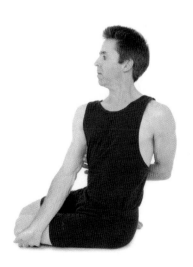

Seated Spinal Twist I

Marichyasana I

Counterpose
- Staff (Dandasana)

Drishti
- Forward
- Downward
- Eyes closed

Physical Benefits
- Tones the abdominal muscles
- Stimulates the digestive, circulatory, and lymphatic systems
- Strengthens and stretches the legs and shoulders
- Massages the kidneys and liver
- Opens the chest and shoulders
- Promotes healthy pituitary gland function

Mental Benefits
- Relieves mild depression
- Reduces stress and anxiety

Contraindications
- High or low blood pressure
- Pregnancy (after the first trimester)
- Insomnia
- Migraine
- Knee or hip injuries (use the gentle variation)

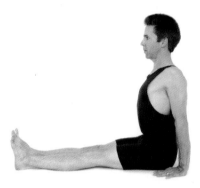

1 Sit in Dandasana (see page 170). Press your hands down into the floor to lengthen your spine.

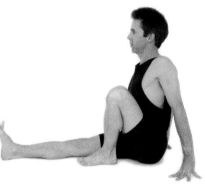

2 Bend your left knee and place your foot on the floor near your right thigh. Distribute your weight evenly between your sitting bones. Place your arms behind you and press your fingertips into the floor. Inhale and extend from the core of your pelvis up through the crown of your head.

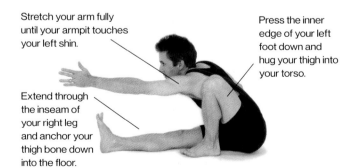

Stretch your arm fully until your armpit touches your left shin.

Press the inner edge of your left foot down and hug your thigh into your torso.

Extend through the inseam of your right leg and anchor your thigh bone down into the floor.

3 Stretch your left arm forward on the inside of your left leg.

4 Internally rotate your left arm and bend the elbow. Wrap your left arm around the outside of your left leg. Bring your right hand around your back and clasp your right wrist with your left hand. Inhale, lengthen up through the sides of your body, and draw your shoulder blades more onto your back. Exhale and twist your torso to the right.

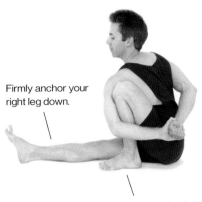

Firmly anchor your right leg down.

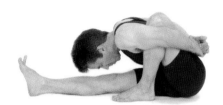

Press the inside of your left foot down to keep both sitting bones rooted into the floor.

5 Inhale and extend from your pelvis through the top of your head. Exhale and bow forward over your right leg. Hold this pose for a few breaths. Release and repeat on the other side.

Gentle Variation

Follow steps 1 through 4 except sit on a folded blanket. Hold a strap between your hands instead of clasping your wrist with your hand.

Other Variation

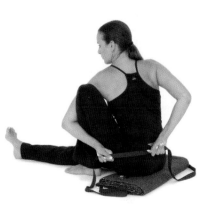

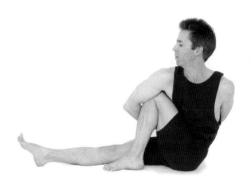

Seated Spinal Twist II

Marichyasana II

Counterpose
- Staff (Dandasana)

Drishti
- Forward
- Downward
- Eyes closed

Physical Benefits
- Tones the abdominal muscles
- Stimulates the digestive, circulatory, and lymphatic systems
- Promotes healthy function of the pituitary gland
- Strengthens and stretches the legs and shoulders
- Massages the kidneys and liver
- Opens the chest and shoulders

Mental Benefits
- Relieves mild depression
- Reduces stress and anxiety

Contraindications
- High or low blood pressure
- Pregnancy (after the first trimester)
- Insomnia
- Migraine
- Knee or hip injuries (use the gentle variation)

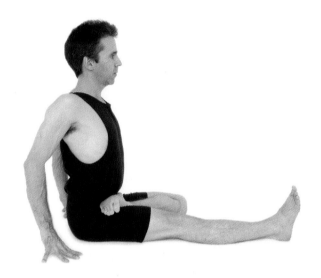

1 Sit with your legs extended (Dandasana, see page 170). Fold your left leg into Half-Lotus by bringing your foot to the top of your right thigh crease. Press your hands into the floor to lengthen your spine.

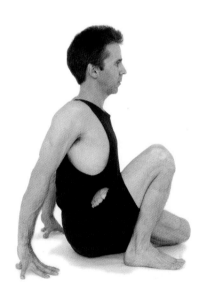

2 Bend your right leg and place your foot near your hips.

3 Inhale and lengthen your spine. Bend at the torso and extend your right arm forward.

Press your left hand into the floor and lengthen the left side of your body.

Stretch your arm fully until the armpit touches your left shin.

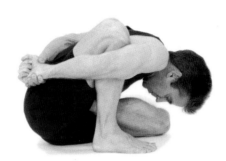

Keep your left foot active by pressing the tops of your toes into your right thigh.

4 Exhale and internally rotate your right arm. Bend the elbow and wrap your arm around the outside of your right shin and thigh. Bring your left arm around your back and clasp your right wrist with your left hand. Inhale, lengthen up through the side of the body, and draw your shoulder blades onto your back. Exhale, bend forward, and bring your head toward your knee.

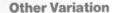

5 Hold this pose for a few breaths. Release, return to step 1, and repeat on the other side.

Gentle Variation

Follow steps 1 through step 5 except sit on a folded blanket, keep one leg extended, and hold a strap between your hands instead of clasping your wrist with your hand.

Other Variation

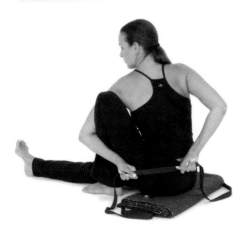

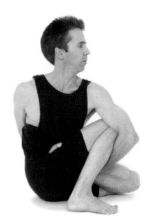

chapter 8

Forward-Bending Postures

Forward bends are calming, soothing to the nervous system, and bring a deeper internal awareness. They open the entire backside of the body, stretching the hamstrings, buttocks, and lower back. They release tension and improve digestions and elimination by massaging the abdominal organs and cleansing the liver and intestines. Seated forward bends increase circulation to the lower extremities and bathe the brain with fresh blood and oxygen.

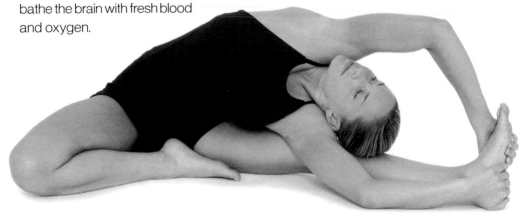

Seated Forward Bend

Paschimottanasana

Counterpose
- Knees-to-Chest (Apanasana)

Drishti
- Closed
- At shins

Physical Benefits
- Stretches the spine, hamstrings, and calves
- Improves digestion
- Stimulates the lymphatic and reproductive systems
- Helps relieve menstrual and menopausal discomfort
- Improves liver, kidney, and colon function
- Alleviates high blood pressure, infertility, and sinusitis
- Reduces fatigue and insomnia

Mental Benefits
- Soothes the nervous system
- Relieves stress, anxiety, and mild depression

Contraindications
- Low back injury (use the gentle variation)
- Asthma
- Pregnancy (use gentle variation keeping legs wide apart)

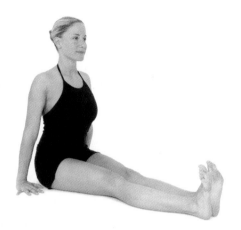

1 Sit with your legs extended. Inhale and press your hands down into the floor to lengthen your spine. Draw your low back inward and upward.

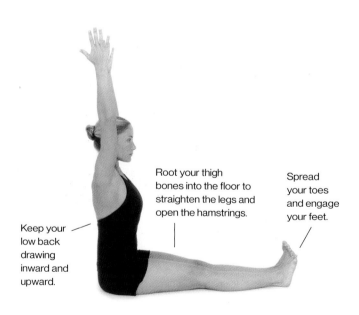

Root your thigh bones into the floor to straighten the legs and open the hamstrings.

Spread your toes and engage your feet.

Keep your low back drawing inward and upward.

2 Inhale and bring your arms up over your head.

3 Exhale, bend forward, and grasp your big toes with your index and middle fingers using a firm grip. Press your big toe forward while resisting back with your fingers.

Pull back muscularly from your hands into your shoulders, drawing your shoulder blades deeply onto your back.

Tilt your pelvis forward, draw your low back in and up creating a concavity in your low back.

Firmly anchor the inner edges of your thighs down and extend from the core of your pelvis out through your feet.

4 Inhale and extend from your low belly up through the top of your head. Slide your hands to the outsides of your feet. Exhale, widen your elbows out, and draw your torso forward toward your feet. Keep your legs actively engaged and straight. Lead with your heart rather than your head.

Keep extending your spine and tilting your sacrum forward.

Press the big-toe sides of your feet forward while drawing the little-toe sides back toward your knees.

Press your hands into the resistance of your feet, draw back muscularly from your hands into your shoulders and actively widen your elbows to draw your torso deeply forward.

Gentle Variation

Follow steps 1 through 3. For tight hamstrings and low back sit on a folded blanket and use a strap around your feet.

Other Variations

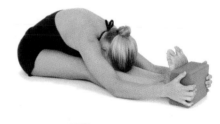

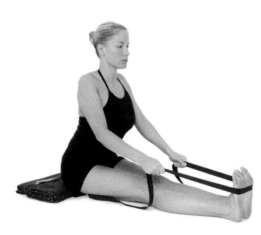

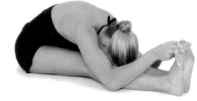

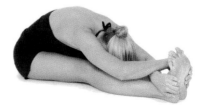

Standing Forward Bend

Uttanasana

Drishti

▷ At shins

▷ Closed

Physical Benefits

▷ Strengthens the feet, knees, and thighs

▷ Stretches the hamstrings and calves

▷ Improves the function of digestive and reproductive systems

▷ Opens the hips and groins

▷ Stimulates the liver, kidneys, and digestive system

▷ Relieves menopausal discomfort, headache, insomnia, and fatigue

▷ Alleviates discomfort from sinusitis

Mental Benefits

▷ Soothes the nervous system

▷ Relieves stress, anxiety, and mild depression

Contraindications

▷ Back injury (keep the knees bent)

▷ Low blood pressure

▷ Pregnancy (widen stance and keep knees bent)

1 Stand in Tadasana with your feet parallel (see page 28).

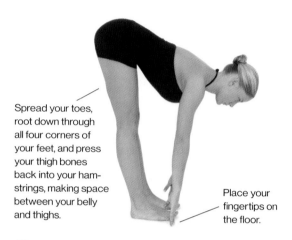

Spread your toes, root down through all four corners of your feet, and press your thigh bones back into your hamstrings, making space between your belly and thighs.

Place your fingertips on the floor.

2 Inhale, stretch your arms up, and extend from your low belly up through your fingertips. Maintaining the length, exhale, bend forward, and touch the floor.

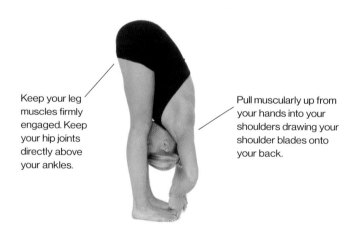

Keep your leg muscles firmly engaged. Keep your hip joints directly above your ankles.

Pull muscularly up from your hands into your shoulders drawing your shoulder blades onto your back.

3 Keeping the space between the belly and thighs, hold your big toes. Use the strength of your inner thighs to widen your sitting bones. Inhale, draw the sides of your waistline up, and root your tailbone down. Exhale and fold your torso deeply forward. Remain for several breaths.

4 **Bring your hands to the backs of your calves.**

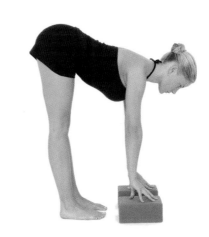

Draw from your hands up into your shoulders to bring the shoulder blades more onto the back.

Press your hands into your calves while actively moving your thighs back against this resistance.

Spread your toes and root all four corners of your feet into the floor.

Gentle Variation

Follow steps 1 through 3. Use a block under your hands to help you keep your legs straight and your lower back concave.

Other Variations

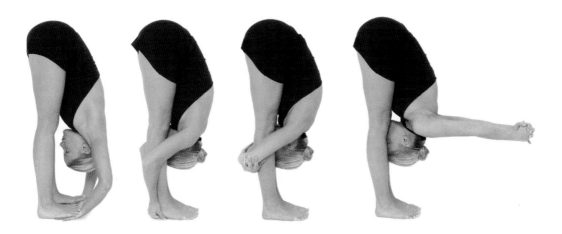

Head-to-Knee Forward Bend

Janu Sirsasana

Counterpose
- Knees-to-Chest (Apanasana)

Drishti
- Forward
- At shins

Physical Benefits
- Opens the chest and lungs
- Stretches the calf, hamstring, and lower back muscles
- Helps relieve menstrual and menopausal discomfort
- Improves digestion
- Increases circulation to the liver, kidneys, and colon
- Alleviates fatigue and headache
- Strengthens the low back

Mental Benefits
- Soothes the nervous system
- Relieves stress, anxiety, and mild depression

Contraindications
- Low blood pressure
- Knee injury (use the gentle variation)
- Asthma

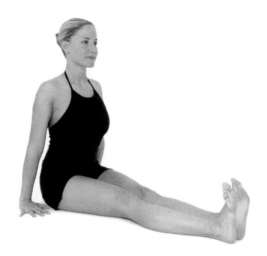

1 Sit with your legs extended. Press your hands into the floor and lengthen your spine upward.

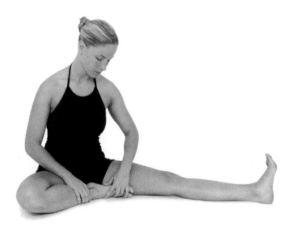

2 Bend your right leg and move your knee out to the right. Place your right heel on the inner edge of your right thigh near the perineum. Rotate your left leg inward so that your knee and foot point straight up.

3 Turn your torso to face your straight leg and extend your arms forward, holding your foot with both hands. Inhale and lengthen from your pelvis up through your head.

Draw muscularly up your arms into your shoulders and bring your shoulder blades deeply onto your back.

Tilt your sacrum forward, draw your low back in and up.

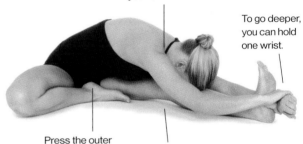

Spread the toes of your left foot and powerfully press your big toe forward into the resistance of your hands.

4 Exhale and extend forward over your left leg, leading with your heart. Reach your hands forward around your left foot. Widen your elbows out, and draw your torso forward. If you are able to keep your spine extended, you can place your forehead on your upper shin. Keep your left leg actively engaged and straight. Press your hands into the resistance of your foot, and actively widen your elbows to draw your torso deeply forward.

Expand into your left waist with your breath and lengthen from your left hip up through your left underarm.

To go deeper, you can hold one wrist.

Press the outer edge of your right foot down into the floor.

Press your left thigh down and extend from the core of your pelvis through the top of your head.

5 Stay in the pose for several good breaths. Release and repeat on the other side.

Gentle Variation

Follow steps 1 through 3. For tight hamstrings and lower back sit on a folded blanket and use a strap around your foot.

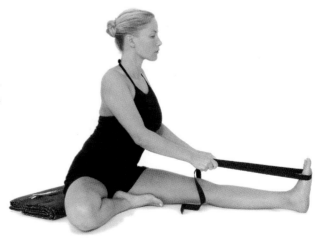

Revolved Head-to-Knee Forward Bend

Parivrtta Janu Sirsasana

Counterpose
▶ Seated Forward Bend
(Paschimottanasana)

Drishti
▶ Closed
▶ Upward
▶ Forward

Physical Benefits
▶ Improves digestion
▶ Stretches the calf,
hamstring, and low back
muscles
▶ Opens the hips, groins, and
shoulders
▶ Opens the musculature and
fascia around the waist, rib
cage, and chest
▶ Stimulates the reproductive
system
▶ Circulates blood to the liver,
colon, and kidneys

Mental Benefits
▶ Soothes the nervous
system
▶ Relieves stress, anxiety, and
mild depression

Contraindications
▶ Low blood pressure
▶ Low back injury
▶ Neck or shoulder injury
▶ Pregnancy (after the first
trimester)

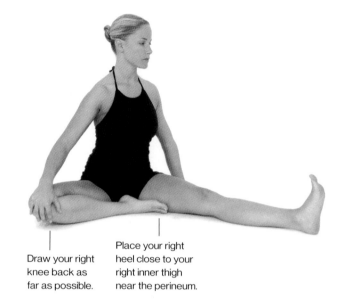

Draw your right
knee back as
far as possible.

Place your right
heel close to your
right inner thigh
near the perineum.

1 Sit with your legs extended. Bend your right
leg and bring your foot to your left thigh with the
knee out to the right. Inhale and lengthen through
the spine. Exhale and turn your torso to face the
straight leg.

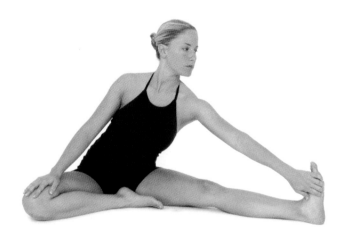

2 Extend your left arm out and hold the inside of
your left foot. Place your right hand on your right
knee.

3 Inhale and extend from your low belly up through the top of your head. Keep the length, exhale, and twist your belly and chest to the right, taking your left shoulder to the inside of your left thigh. Reach up with your right arm to hold the outside of your left foot.

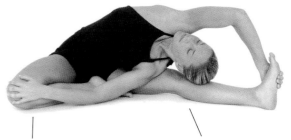

Press your left hand on your right knee to facilitate a deeper twist.

Press your left thigh bone down and extend from the core of your pelvis out through your feet.

4 Bring your left arm around to clasp the inside of your left foot, drawing your left shoulder even further inside your left thigh. With each inhale extend from your low belly through your head. With each exhale twist more deeply. Hold for several breaths then release and repeat on the other side.

Twist your torso upward resting the back of your head on your left leg.

Widen your elbows apart.

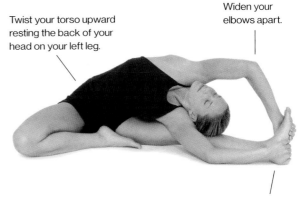

Turn your left hand so that the thumb is facing downward.

Gentle Variation

Perform steps 1 and 2. Place your left hand on your left shin and stretch your right hand up toward the ceiling.

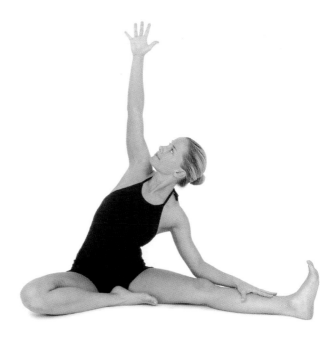

Open-Angle

Upavistha Konasana

Counterpose
▶ Knees-to-Chest (Apanasana)

Drishti
▶ Forward
▶ On the floor, directly under nose

Physical Benefits
▶ Strengthens the low back
▶ Lengthens the spine
▶ Opens the hips, groin, and shoulders
▶ Stretches the hamstrings, calves, and inner thighs
▶ Stimulates digestive and reproductive systems
▶ Increases circulation to liver and kidneys

Mental Benefits
▶ Soothes the nervous system
▶ Relieves stress, anxiety, and mild depression

Contraindications
▶ Low blood pressure
▶ Low back injury
▶ Groin or hamstring injury

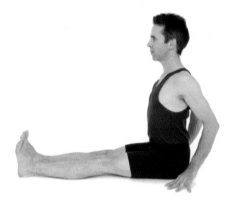

1 **Sit with your legs extended. Press your fingertips into the ground and lengthen your spine upward.**

Tilt your sacrum forward to create a natural curve in your low back and extend from the core of your pelvis up through the top of your head.

Bring your hands behind your back and press your fingertips down.

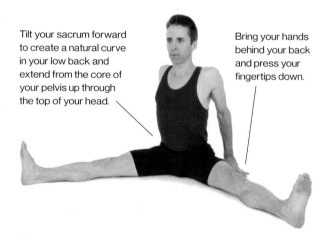

2 **Widen your legs and rotate them inward so that your feet and knees point straight up. Manually rotate the flesh of your thighs inward (inseam moves downward) with your hands and widen your pelvic floor by moving your buttocks flesh out to the side and back. Spread your toes.**

3 Maintain the curve in your low back. Inhale, elongate your spine, and bring your hands forward onto your fingertips. Firmly ground the inseams of your thighs into the floor; extend from your low belly out through your legs and spread your toes.

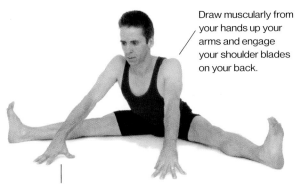

Draw muscularly from your hands up your arms and engage your shoulder blades on your back.

Press your fingertips down and drag your hands back toward your body against the resistance of the floor.

4 Inhale and lengthen from the core of your pelvis up through the crown of your head. Exhale, bend your elbows out to the sides, and bring your torso forward, leading with your heart. If you are able to keep your spine extended, you can rest your forehead on the ground. Stay in the pose for several breaths, then release.

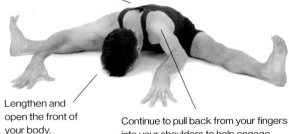

Lift your elbows and the fronts of your shoulders and draw your shoulder blades more deeply onto your back.

Lengthen and open the front of your body.

Continue to pull back from your fingers into your shoulders to help engage your shoulder blades on your back.

Gentle Variation

Follow steps 1 through 4. For tight hamstrings or low back use a folded blanket under your hips.

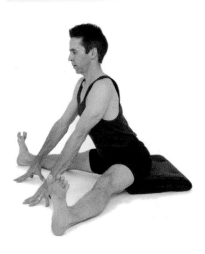

Other Variations

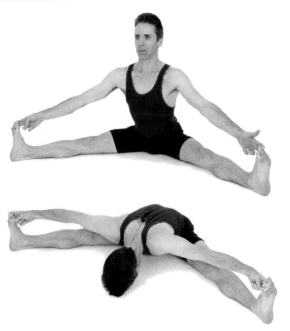

145

Side Open-Angle

Parsva Upavistha Konasana

Drishti
- Forward
- At knee or shin

Physical Benefits
- Improves digestion
- Stretches the calf, hamstring, and low back muscles
- Strengthens the low back
- Promotes spinal flexibility
- Opens musculature and fascia around the waist and rib cage
- Opens the hips, groin, and shoulders
- Stimulates the reproductive system
- Increases circulation to the liver and kidneys

Mental Benefits
- Soothes the nervous system
- Relieves stress, anxiety, and mild depression

Contraindications
- Low blood pressure
- Low back injury (use the gentle variation)

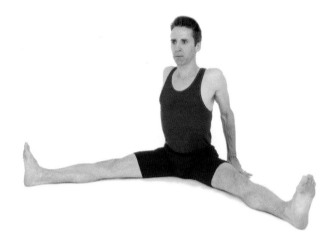

1 Sit with your legs extended. Widen your legs apart to approximately 90 degrees and inwardly rotate them so that your feet and knees point straight up. Manually widen your pelvic floor by moving your buttocks flesh out to the side and back. Spread your toes. Bring your hands behind you and firmly press the fingertips down. Tilt your pelvis forward to create a natural curve in the low back.

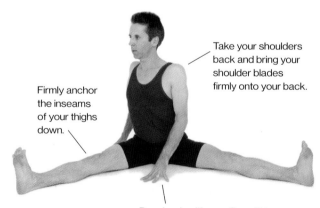

Take your shoulders back and bring your shoulder blades firmly onto your back.

Firmly anchor the inseams of your thighs down.

Drag back with your fingertips against the resistance of the floor.

2 Place your fingertips on either side of your right leg and turn your torso to the right. Exhale and root your thighs and sitting bones down. Inhale, lengthen from your low belly through your head, and shift your belly, lungs, and heart to the right. Pull back toward your body with your hands.

3 Exhale, extend forward over your right leg, and hold your right foot with both hands.

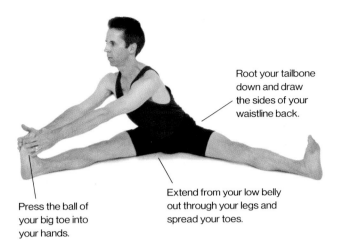

Root your tailbone down and draw the sides of your waistline back.

Press the ball of your big toe into your hands.

Extend from your low belly out through your legs and spread your toes.

4 Inhale and extend from your low belly up through your head. Exhale and extend forward over your leg, leading with your heart. If you are able to keep your spine extended, you can bring your forehead toward your upper shin. Stay in the pose for several breaths. Release and repeat on the other side.

Lift your elbows and the fronts of your shoulders to help you draw your shoulder blades more deeply onto your back.

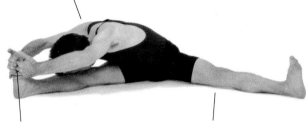

Actively spread your toes and press your foot into your hands. Use the resistance of your foot and pull back with your hands to engage the muscles all the way up the arms and into the shoulders.

Press your thigh bones down and powerfully extend out through your legs.

Gentle Variation
Follow steps 1 through 3. For tight hamstrings and low back sit on a folded blanket and use a strap around your foot.

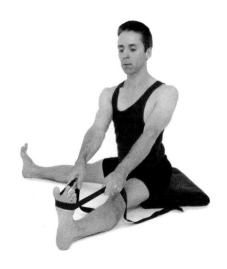

147

Three-Limb Intense Stretch

Triang Mukaikapada Paschimottanasana

Counterpose

▶ Downward-Facing Dog
(Adho Mukha Svanasana)

Drishti

▶ Forward

▶ On shin or kneecap

Physical Benefits

▶ Stretches the spine,
hamstrings, and calves

▶ Helps relieve menstrual and
menopausal discomfort

▶ Enhances liver, kidney, and
colon function

▶ Assists with symptoms
of high blood pressure,
infertility, and sinusitis

▶ Reduces fatigue

▶ Stimulates thyroid and
parathyroid activity

Mental Benefits

▶ Soothes the nervous
system

▶ Relieves stress, anxiety, and
mild depression

Contraindications

▶ Knee or low back injury (use
the gentle variation)

▶ Asthma

▶ Pregnancy

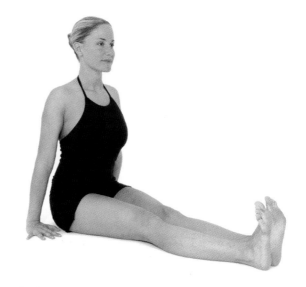

1 Sit with your legs extended. Press your hands into the floor and lengthen your spine upward.

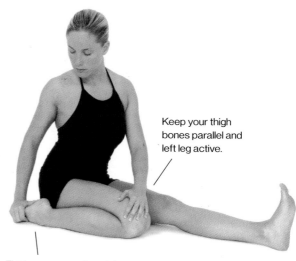

Keep your thigh
bones parallel and
left leg active.

Firmly press your toes into
the floor, and hug your right
ankle in toward your hip.

2 Bend your right leg and place your ankle by the side of your right hip. Point your right foot straight back. Manually widen your hip flesh to the sides and distribute your weight evenly between your right and left buttocks.

148

3 Extend your arms forward and hold the sides of your left foot with both hands. Inhale and extend from your low belly up through your head.

Draw your lower back in and up.

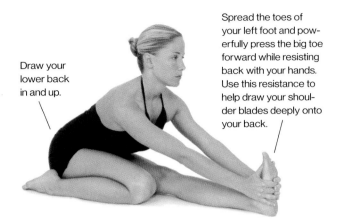

Spread the toes of your left foot and powerfully press the big toe forward while resisting back with your hands. Use this resistance to help draw your shoulder blades deeply onto your back.

4 Exhale, widen your elbows out to the sides, and extend your torso forward, leading with your heart. Keep your left leg actively engaged and straight. If you are able to keep your spine extended, you can touch your head to your shin.

Keep your right sitting bone grounded to counter the tendency for your right hip to lift.

Anchor the inseam of your left leg down and extend from your low belly out through your foot.

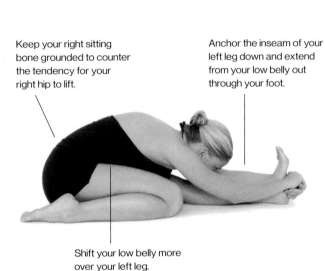

Shift your low belly more over your left leg.

Gentle Variation

Follow steps 1 through 4. To help keep your hips level use a folded blanket under the straight-leg hip and use a strap around your foot.

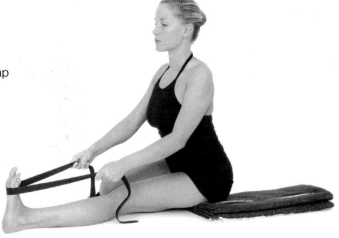

Garland

Malasana

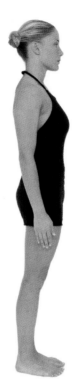

Counterpose
▷ Staff (Dandasana)

Drishti
▷ Forward

Physical Benefits
▷ Increases circulation to digestive system
▷ Opens the hips
▷ Relieves sciatica
▷ Improves balance
▷ Strengthens the arches of the feet and ankles
▷ Helps relieve menstrual discomfort
▷ Alleviates low back pain
▷ Helps relieve constipation

Mental Benefits
▷ Relieves stress, anxiety, and mild depression
▷ Creates poise
▷ Cultivates focus

Contraindications
▷ Ankle or knee injury
▷ Vertigo
▷ High blood pressure (broaden your stance)

1 Stand in Tadasana with the inner edges of your feet touching (see page 28).

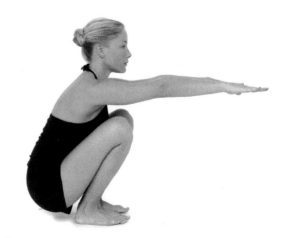

2 Bring your arms parallel with the floor to help with balance. With your feet together and flat on the ground, exhale and squat down keeping your hips off the floor.

3 Widen your knees apart and lean forward between them. Stretch your arms forward until your upper arms touch the insides of your knees and bring your hands into a prayer position.

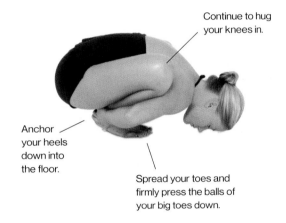

Root your tailbone down and extend from the core of your pelvis up through the crown of your head.

Press your hands together and widen your elbows out against the resistance of your knees drawing in.

Press the inner edges of your feet down and hug your knees into your upper arms.

4 Inhale, reach back with your hands, and hold your heels. Exhale and bring your head to the ground. Hold this pose for a few breaths, then release.

Continue to hug your knees in.

Anchor your heels down into the floor.

Spread your toes and firmly press the balls of your big toes down.

Gentle Variation

Follow steps 1 through 3, but place a folded blanket under your heels.

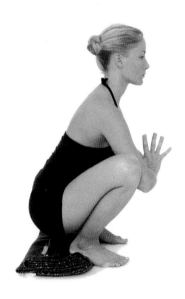

Splits

Hanumanasana

Counterpose
▶ Downward-Facing Dog (Adho Mukha Svanasana)

Drishti
▶ Forward
▶ Upward

Physical Benefits
▶ Strengthens and tones thighs and hamstrings
▶ Opens the hips and groin and psoas muscles
▶ Improves circulation
▶ Prevents varicose veins
▶ Stimulates digestive, lymphatic, and reproductive systems
▶ Stimulates abdominal organs
▶ Prevents and relieves symptoms of sciatica and hernia
▶ Improves balance

Mental Benefits
▶ Calms the mind
▶ Reduces stress, mild depression, and anxiety

Contraindications
▶ Groin injury
▶ Knee or hamstring injury
▶ High or low blood pressure (do not raise hands overhead)

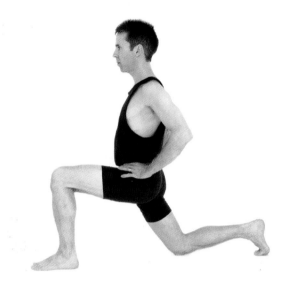

1 Kneel on the floor. Take a big step forward with your left leg and curl the toes of the back foot under.

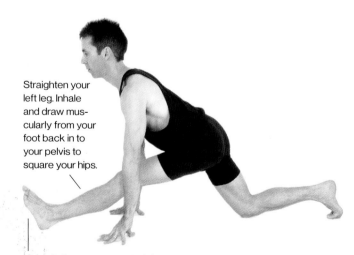

Straighten your left leg. Inhale and draw muscularly from your foot back in to your pelvis to square your hips.

Maintain the engagement of the foot and calf muscles by spreading your toes and pressing through the ball of the big toe.

2 Place your fingertips on the floor.

3 Walk your hands back closer to your hips. Exhale, tuck your tailbone down and under, and extend from the core of your pelvis out through both legs.

Keep the muscles of both legs engaged and lower your pelvis to the floor.

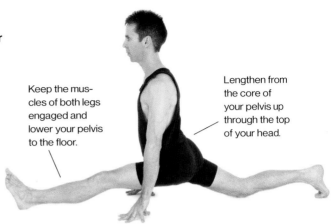

Lengthen from the core of your pelvis up through the top of your head.

4 Inhale and draw from the feet into the pelvis again. Exhale, tuck your tailbone under again and extend from your pelvis out through the bones of the legs as you bring your hips all the way to the floor. Extend fully through your legs. Raise your arms over your head.

5 Release and repeat on the other side.

Vibrantly extend your arms up and open your fingers enthusiastically.

Maintain a strong inner spiral in your back leg by curling the toes of your back foot under. The weight of your body should rest on the front of your right thigh.

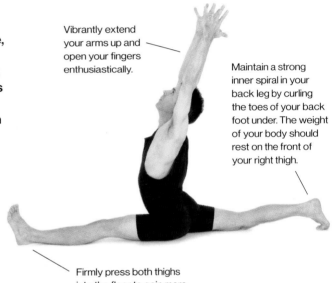

Firmly press both thighs into the floor to gain more lift in your torso.

Gentle Variation

Follow steps 1 through 4. Place your hands on blocks placed on either side of your thighs and keep your torso lifted and your spine straight.

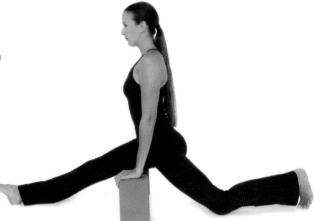

chapter 9

Sitting Postures

Sitting and meditation postures are generally calming and nurturing, although some produce significant opening of the hip and require greater effort. They promote vitality when practiced with proper alignment of the spine and pelvis. They improve circulation, reduce fatigue, center the mind, and soothe the nervous system. Sitting and meditation poses can be done at any time. Meditation poses should be practiced daily in conjunction with your asana practice.

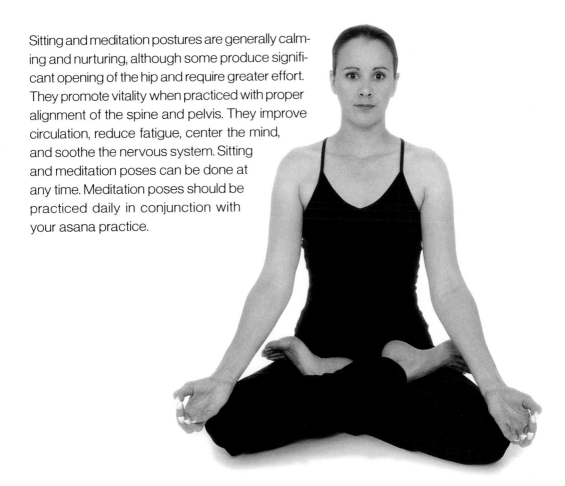

Lotus

Padmasana

Counterpose
- Staff (Dandasana)

Drishti
- Forward
- Eyes closed

Physical Benefits
- Opens the hips
- Increases knee flexibility and lubricates the knee joints
- Prevents arthritis and osteoporosis
- Tones abdominal organs
- Promotes proper digestive system functions

Mental Benefits
- Focuses the mind
- Reduces stress
- Brings mental clarity

Contraindications
- Low back, hip, knee, or ankle injury (use the gentle variation)

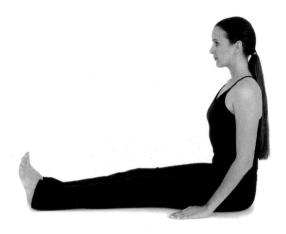

1 Sit with your legs extended (Dandasana, page 170) and lengthen your spine from the tailbone up through the crown of your head.

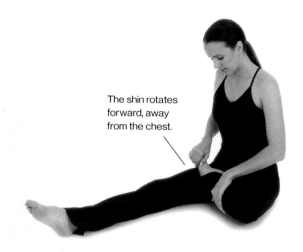

The shin rotates forward, away from the chest.

2 Draw one heel to your navel, rotate your leg and foot outward, and place the top of your foot on top of your out-stretched thigh at the hip crease.

3 Draw your other heel to your navel, rotate your leg and foot outward, and place the top of your foot on top of your opposite thigh at the hip crease. Use your hands to broaden the base of your pelvic floor; that is, rotate your thighs and hips inward, one at a time, as you widen them out to the sides.

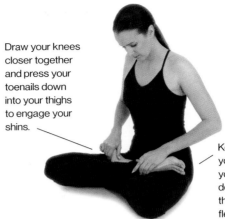

Draw your knees closer together and press your toenails down into your thighs to engage your shins.

Keep the width in your pelvic floor as you root the tailbone down and under so that the buttocks flesh flows down in back.

4 Inhale deeply and extend from your low belly up through the top of your head. Lengthen up through the sides of your body, draw your shoulders back, and slide your shoulder blades down your back. Soften into the pose by relaxing your breath. Remain in the pose as long as desired.

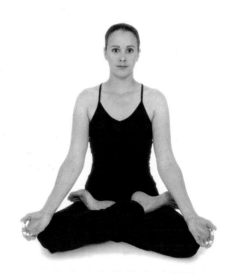

Gentle Variation
Follow steps 1 through 4 except place only one foot in Lotus.

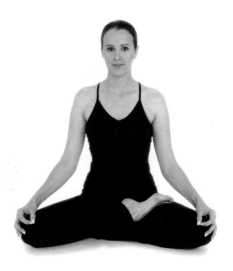

Looking Within

Padmasana With Sanmukhi Mudra

Counterpose
▶ Staff (Dandasana)

Drishti
▶ Eyes closed

Physical Benefits
▶ Calms the nervous system

Mental Benefits
▶ Focuses the mind
▶ Reduces stress
▶ Brings mental clarity
▶ Blocks sensory input and removes external distractions

Contraindications
▶ Glaucoma
▶ Hearing aids (do not restrict ear canal while wearing)
▶ Corneal disease (place fingertips gently on eyelids instead of applying pressure)

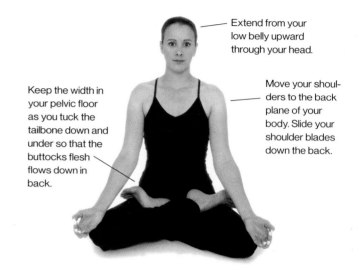

Extend from your low belly upward through your head.

Move your shoulders to the back plane of your body. Slide your shoulder blades down the back.

Keep the width in your pelvic floor as you tuck the tailbone down and under so that the buttocks flesh flows down in back.

1 Begin in Lotus (see page 156). Use your hands to broaden the base of your pelvic floor; that is, rotate your thighs and hips inward, one at a time, as you widen them out to the sides.

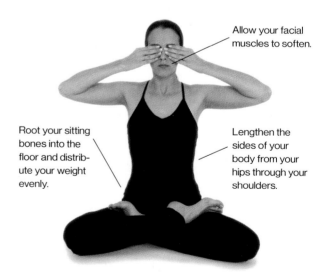

Allow your facial muscles to soften.

Root your sitting bones into the floor and distribute your weight evenly.

Lengthen the sides of your body from your hips through your shoulders.

2 Rest your fingers on your eyelids, applying slight pressure; continue with deep, even breathing through your nose.

3 If desired, begin to close off your senses, one by one, going deeper into yourself. Place your thumbs in your ears to cut off external sounds. Place your first and second fingers on your eyes, distributing the gentle pressure evenly. Allow your index fingers to softly pull your eyelids toward your eyebrows as the second fingers draw the eyelids closed. Shut both corners of your eyes. Use your third fingers to press your nostrils, and place your pinky fingers on your top lip to gauge rhythm of your breath.

4 When ready, lower your hands and release your legs.

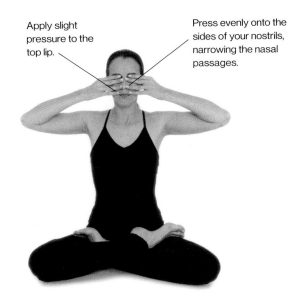

Apply slight pressure to the top lip.

Press evenly onto the sides of your nostrils, narrowing the nasal passages.

Gentle Variation

Sit in Siddhasana variation (see page 176) and follow steps 2 through 4.

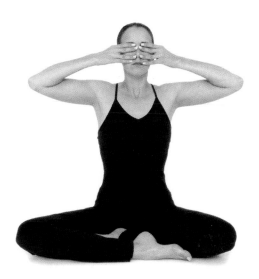

Baby Cradle

Counterpose
▷ Staff (Dandasana)

Drishti
▷ Forward

Physical Benefits
▷ Stretches the thighs, hamstrings, and calf muscles
▷ Creates proper engagement of the hamstrings
▷ Improves digestion
▷ Massages the abdominal muscles
▷ Stimulates the colon, liver, and kidneys
▷ Opens the pelvic region
▷ Stimulates the reproductive and digestive systems

Mental Benefits
▷ Soothes the nervous system
▷ Develops mental focus
▷ Calms the mind

Contraindication
▷ Knee or hip injury

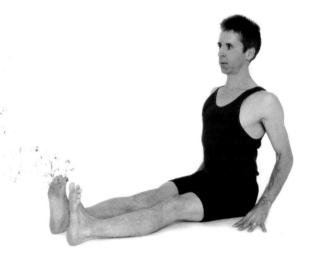

1 Sit with your legs extended. Press your hands into the floor to lengthen your spine.

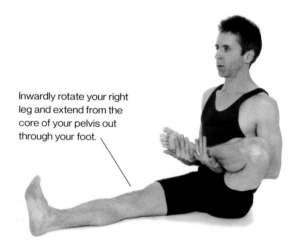

Inwardly rotate your right leg and extend from the core of your pelvis out through your foot.

2 Bend your left leg and draw your knee out to the side. Bring your hands underneath your leg, cradling your foot and lower shin.

3 Bring your left leg up and parallel to the floor.

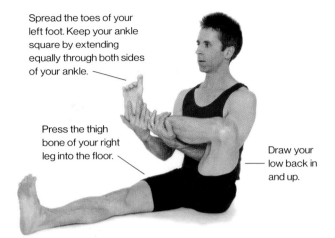

Spread the toes of your left foot. Keep your ankle square by extending equally through both sides of your ankle.

Press the thigh bone of your right leg into the floor.

Draw your low back in and up.

4 Cradle your left foot in the elbow of your right arm. Wrap your left arm around the outside of your left knee and lower leg. Clasp your right wrist with your left hand. Inhale, and move your left knee slightly away from your body. Exhale, and draw your shin and foot in toward your torso.

5 Release and repeat on the other side.

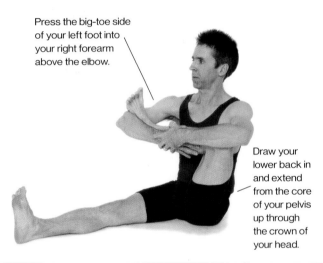

Press the big-toe side of your left foot into your right forearm above the elbow.

Draw your lower back in and extend from the core of your pelvis up through the crown of your head.

Gentle Variation

Bend the knee of your bottom leg and draw the foot in close to your body.

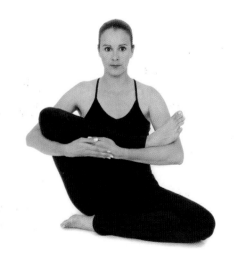

Hero

Virasana

Counterposes

▷ Downward-Facing Dog (Adho Mukha Svanasana)

▷ Seated Forward Bend (Paschimottanasana)

Drishti

▷ At ceiling

▷ Eyes closed

Physical Benefits

▷ Opens the lower back

▷ Improves the health and function of the hip, knee, and ankle joints

▷ Stimulates thyroid and parathyroid productivity

▷ Helps relieve menopausal discomfort

▷ Helps relieve high blood pressure

Mental Benefits

▷ Creates a feeling of grounding and stability

▷ Calms the mind

Contraindications

▷ Knee or ankle injury (use the gentle variation)

▷ Arthritis (use the gentle variation)

▷ Heart disease

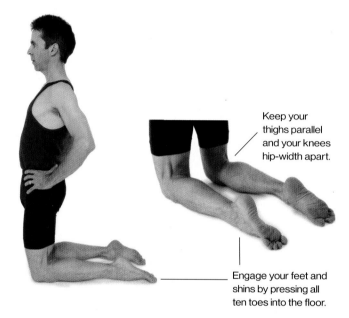

Keep your thighs parallel and your knees hip-width apart.

Engage your feet and shins by pressing all ten toes into the floor.

1 Kneel on the floor.

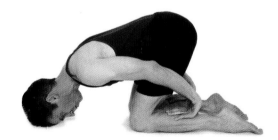

2 Bring your forehead to the floor and place your hands on your calves behind your knees. Press your fingers into your calves with a steady pressure and slide your hands down toward your ankles to flatten your calves evenly.

3 Bring your buttocks to the floor and rest your hands on your thighs. Root your sitting bones down and lengthen from the core of your pelvis up through the crown of your head. Maintain a natural curve in your spine.

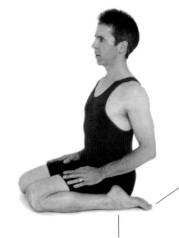

Keep pressing your toes into the floor and hug your ankles in toward your hips.

Keep your ankles by the sides of your hips.

Gentle Variation

Follow steps 1 through 3 except sit on a folded blanket or bolster to elevate your hips.

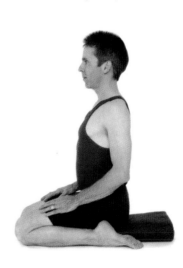

Other Variations

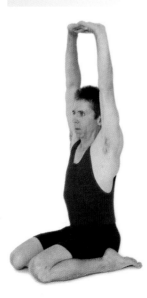

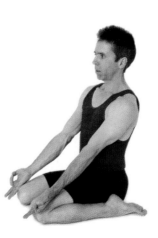

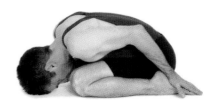

Kneeling Pose

Bhujrasana

Counterpose
- Staff (Dandasana)

Drishti
- Forward

Physical Benefits
- Stimulates circulation
- Energizes the thighs, calves, and ankles
- Aligns the spine
- Stretches the quadriceps
- Opens ankle, knee, and hip joints

Mental Benefits
- Calms the mind
- Soothes the nervous system

Contraindications
- Knee injury
- Ankle injury

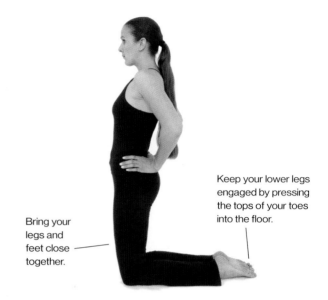

Bring your legs and feet close together.

Keep your lower legs engaged by pressing the tops of your toes into the floor.

1 **Kneel on the floor.**

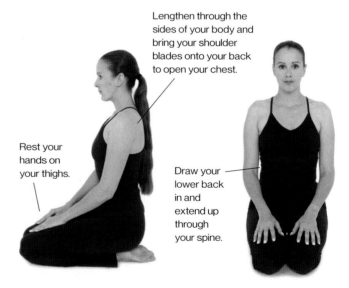

Lengthen through the sides of your body and bring your shoulder blades onto your back to open your chest.

Rest your hands on your thighs.

Draw your lower back in and extend up through your spine.

Front view

2 **Sit down on your heels.**

Gentle Variation

Follow steps 1 through 2. Place
a bolster or folded blankets
underneath your hips.

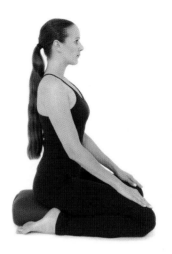

Other Variation

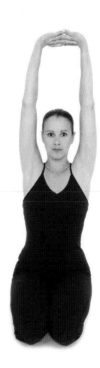

Lion

Simhasana

Counterpose
- Child's Pose (Balasana)

Drishti
- Forward
- Upward

Physical Benefits
- Relieves jaw tension
- Exercises the facial muscles
- Improves blood flow to the brain
- Increases circulation to the eyes and throat
- Clears nasal and ear passages
- Helps relieve sinusitis
- Increases lung capacity
- Relieves dry or sore throats

Mental Benefits
- Reduces stress, mild depression, and anxiety

Contraindications
- Ankle or knee injury (see gentle variation)
- Asthma
- Glaucoma
- Temporomandibular joint syndrome (TMJ)

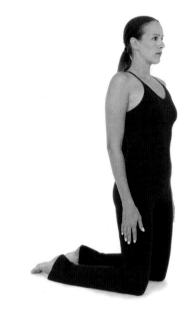

1 Kneel on the floor.

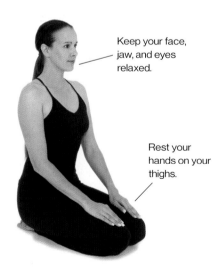

Keep your face, jaw, and eyes relaxed.

Rest your hands on your thighs.

2 Point your toes and sit back on your heels.

3 Lean your torso forward and place your fingertips on the floor. Inhale deeply. On your next exhalation, let out an audible and long sigh. Repeat three times, then relax.

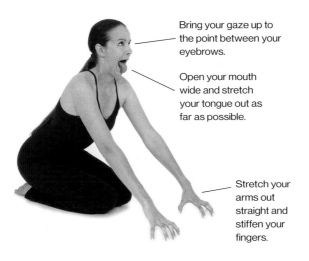

Bring your gaze up to the point between your eyebrows.

Open your mouth wide and stretch your tongue out as far as possible.

Stretch your arms out straight and stiffen your fingers.

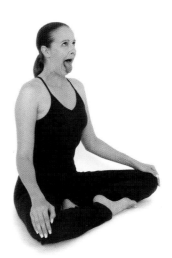

Gentle Variation

Sit in a comfortable cross-legged position then follow step 3.

Other Variations

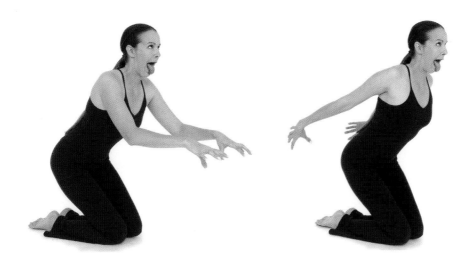

Cow Face

Gomukhasana

Counterpose
- Staff (Dandasana)

Drishti
- Forward
- Closed

Physical Benefits
- Opens the knee, ankle, and shoulder joints
- Stretches the thighs, chest, and arms
- Opens the chest enabling deeper breathing
- Stretches the entire back
- Tones the abdominal muscles and lower back

Mental Benefits
- Improves focus
- Reduces stress, mild depression, and anxiety

Contraindications
- Shoulder injury
- Ankle, knee, or hip injury (use the gentle variation)

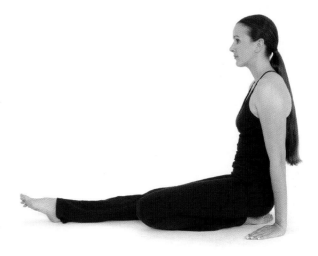

1 Sit with your legs extended. Press your hands into the floor and raise your buttocks. Bend your left leg back and sit on your left foot.

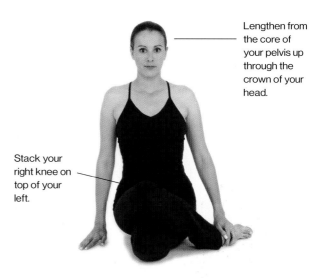

Lengthen from the core of your pelvis up through the crown of your head.

Stack your right knee on top of your left.

2 Bend your right leg and bring your right thigh on top of your left.

3 Either maintain the position of your left foot or lift your hips and move your foot outside your right hip to bring both hips to the floor. Raise your left arm over your head and bend your elbow, resting your hand on your upper back. Bend your right arm, bring the forearm up your back, and clasp your hands together.

4 Release and repeat on the other side.

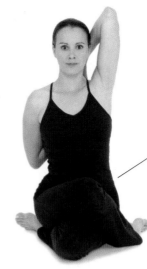

Fully extend your spine from the tailbone up through the crown of your head.

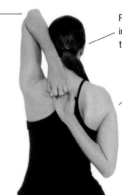

Draw muscularly from your left elbow back into your armpit hollowing your armpit back. Keeping the engagement, extend your elbow higher.

Press your head back into your arm keeping the chest open.

Lengthen up through the right side of your body and draw the right shoulder back.

Back view of hand clasp

Gentle Variation

Follow the instructions in steps 1 through 3. At step 3 place a bolster or folded blanket under your hips. Use a strap between your hands.

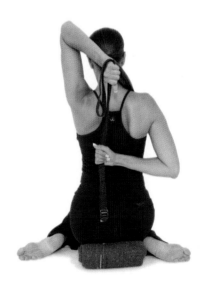

169

Staff Pose

Dandasana

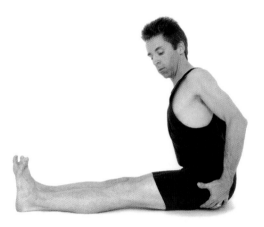

Counterpose
▷ Seated Forward Bend
(Paschimottanasana)

Drishti
▷ Forward

Physical Benefits
▷ Tones abdominal muscles
▷ Increases circulation
▷ Opens the chest
▷ Strengthens legs, torso,
arms, and spine
▷ Improves muscular
endurance of legs and
lumbar spine

Mental Benefits
▷ Creates focus
▷ Reduces stress

Contraindications
▷ None

1 Sit with your legs extended. Widen the pelvic
floor by rotating your legs inward (the inseam of
the leg moves down). Rotate the legs inward by
firmly holding the inside of your left thigh with your
right hand and the outside of your left hip with
your left hand. Rotate your thigh muscles inwardly
by drawing the inseam of the thigh down and the
outer hip up as you lean slightly to the right. Simultaneously widen the thigh and hip out to the left
side. Repeat on your right leg.

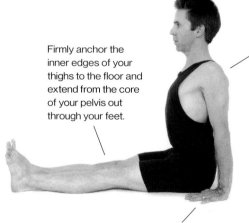

Firmly anchor the
inner edges of your
thighs to the floor and
extend from the core
of your pelvis out
through your feet.

Bring your
shoulder
blades
more onto
your back
to open the
chest.

Exhale, press your hands
down, and lengthen the sides
of your body upward.

2 Press your hands into the floor to lengthen
your spine.

Gentle Variation

Follow steps 1 and 2, but place a bolster or folded blankets under your hips.

Yoga Sealing Pose

Yoga Mudrasana

Counterpose
▷ Staff (Dandasana)

Drishti
▷ Forward
▷ Upward

Physical Benefits
▷ Opens hips and chest
▷ Increases knee flexibility
▷ Prevents arthritis and osteoporosis
▷ Promotes digestive and reproductive system health
▷ Stretches shoulders
▷ Stimulates intestines, colon, and liver
▷ Relieves sciatica and menstrual discomfort

Mental Benefits
▷ Calms the mind
▷ Reduces stress

Contraindications
▷ High or low blood pressure (do not bend forward)
▷ Pregnancy (after the first trimester; do not bend forward)
▷ Groin or shoulder injury
▷ Knee or hip injury

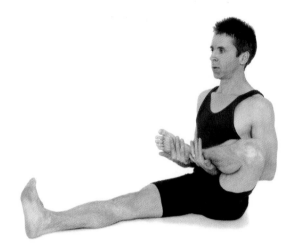

1 Sit with your legs extended. Bend your left leg and bring your hands underneath your leg, cradling the foot and lower shin.

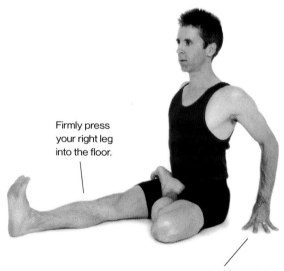

Firmly press your right leg into the floor.

Place your hands behind your back and press your fingertips into the floor to lengthen your spine.

2 Fold your left leg into Half-Lotus by bringing your foot to the top of your right thigh crease.

3 Bend your right leg and hold your right foot and ankle. Come to the full lotus pose by bringing your right foot up to the crease of your left thigh. Exhale, press your hands down, and extend from the core of your pelvis up through the crown of your head. Maintain a natural curve in your spine.

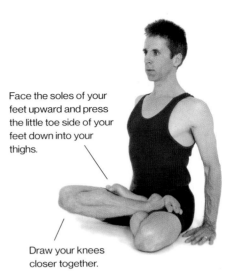

Face the soles of your feet upward and press the little toe side of your feet down into your thighs.

Draw your knees closer together.

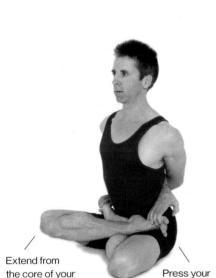

Extend from the core of your pelvis out through your knees.

Press your toes down into your thighs.

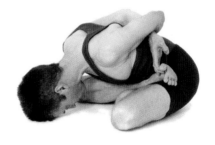

4 Exhale and bring your right arm behind your back and grab your big toe. Take a breath in, lean your torso forward, exhale, swing your left arm around behind your back, and grab the other big toe.

5 Curl your head back, look up and take a few breaths (see variation posture). Exhale and bend forward, resting your forehead on the floor. Release and repeat on the other side.

Other Variation

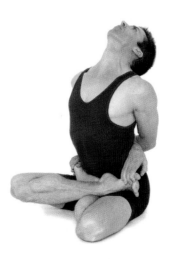

Heron

Krounchasana

Counterpose
- Staff (Dandasana)

Drishti
- Forward
- At big toe

Physical Benefits
- Stretches shoulders, chest, back, and hamstrings
- Improves digestion
- Stimulates reproductive and lymphatic system
- Improves liver, kidney, uterus, and ovary function
- Relieves menstrual and menopausal discomfort
- Relieves backache and fatigue

Mental Benefits
- Calms the mind
- Reduces stress, mild depression, and anxiety

Contraindications
- Insomnia
- Asthma
- Pregnancy (after the first trimester)
- Knee or ankle injuries
- Hip injuries (use a folded blanket under hip for support)

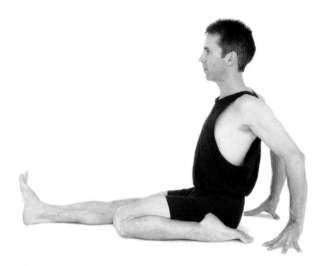

1 Sit with your legs extended. Bend your left leg and rest your ankle by the side of your hip. Keep your knees parallel. Press your hands into the floor. Root your sitting bones down into the floor and lengthen up through the spine.

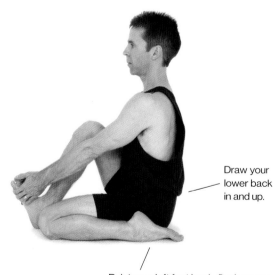

Draw your lower back in and up.

Point your left foot back, firmly press your toes into the floor, and hug your left ankle in toward your hip.

2 Bend your right knee and hold your foot with both hands.

174

3 Exhale and straighten your right leg up. Draw from your hands back through your arms to your shoulders, and hollow your armpits. Bring your shoulder blades onto your back. Maintain this pose for a few breaths.

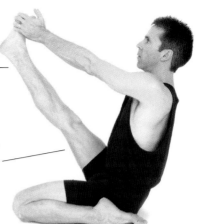

Fully extend from the core of your pelvis out through your right leg.

Press your right thigh bone away from your belly to engage the hamstring muscle.

4 Keep pressing your right thigh away from your belly, exhale, and draw your right shin in toward your body while moving your torso and head forward.

5 Release and repeat on the other side.

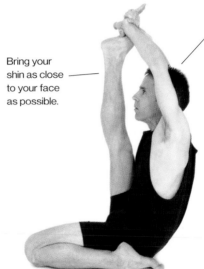

Bring your shin as close to your face as possible.

Widen your elbows away from each other to draw your leg in deeper.

Gentle Variation
Follow only steps 1 through 3. Use a strap across the sole of your foot.

Sage

Siddhasana

Counterpose
▷ Staff (Dandasana)

Drishti
▷ Forward
▷ Eyes closed

Physical Benefits
▷ Increases blood circulation in the lower spine
▷ Tones abdominal organs through breathing action
▷ Elongates the spine
▷ Opens the hips
▷ Strengthens the low and middle back
▷ Calms the nervous system

Mental Benefits
▷ Focuses the mind
▷ Reduces stress
▷ Brings mental clarity

Contraindications
▷ Low back, hip, knee, or ankle injury (use the gentle variation)

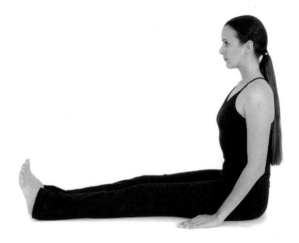

1 Sit with your legs extended (Dandasana, page 170) as you lengthen your spine from the tailbone up through the crown of your head.

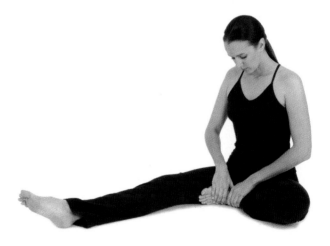

2 Bring the sole of your left foot to the inner edge of your right thigh with the heel in toward the perineum.

3 Gently bend your right leg and draw your heel in toward your body. Place the top of your right foot and ankle onto the left calf muscle. Use your hands to broaden the base of your pelvic floor; that is, rotate your thighs and hips inward, one at a time, as you widen them out to the sides.

Keep the width in your pelvic floor as you tuck your tailbone down and under so that the buttocks flesh flows down in back.

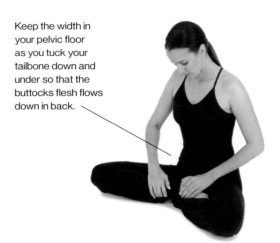

4 Rest your palms, face up, on your thighs, with your thumb and index fingers touching. Exhale and root down into the floor with your sitting bones. Let your legs and pelvis be heavy. Inhale, and extend from the core of your low belly up through the crown of your head. Remain in the pose as long as desired.

Close your eyes, soften your breath, and focus inwardly.

Lengthen up through your sides, draw your shoulder blades onto your back and take them down your back toward your waist.

Continue to tuck your tailbone down and draw your navel in and up.

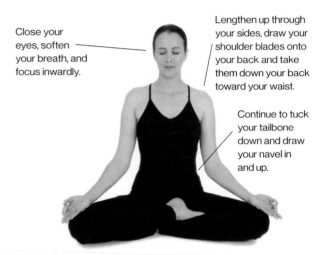

Gentle Variation

For low back tightness, sit on the edge of a folded blanket throughout steps 1 to 4.

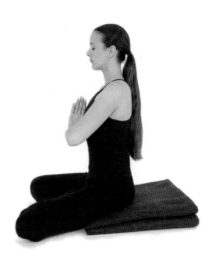

Other Variations—
Hand Mudras

A *mudra* is a hand gesture that completes an energy circuit in the body and mind. They help to create a calming effect and to encourage different mental focus. More information is available in chapter 1, pages 25 to 26.

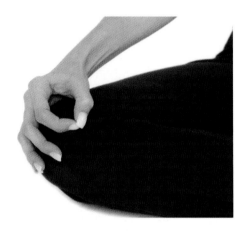

Gyana mudra

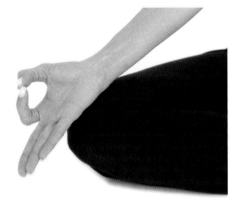

Gyana mudra

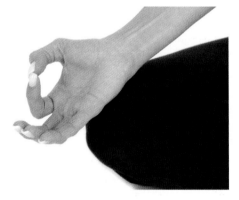

Gyana mudra

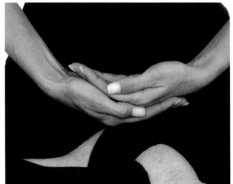

Dhyana mudra

chapter 10

Reclining and Relaxation Postures

Reclining poses are generally done as a cool down at the end of a practice. They reduce fatigue, increase mental clarity, and open spaces within the body that are generally closed by tension. Each of the reclining poses in this chapter increases flexibility through the groins and hips, stimulates digestion and elimination, and strengthens and stretches the lower back and legs.

Relaxation poses soothe and balance the nervous system, offering the body rest from physical activity. Child's pose is used throughout a practice whenever a rest is needed. Corpse pose is the quintessential restorative pose. It is typically performed at the end of a practice for deep relaxation and rejuvenation. The corpse pose is often regarded as the most difficult of poses because it requires being still and receptive.

It is important to take time in both reclining and relaxation poses to breathe and completely embrace the sensations experienced when practicing them.

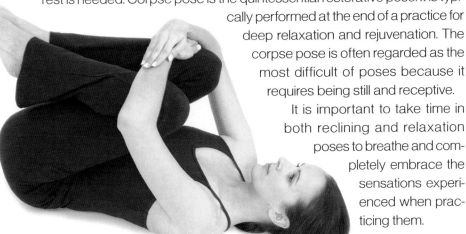

Knees-to-Chest

Apanasana

Counterpose
▸ Corpse (Savasana)

Drishti
▸ Eyes closed
▸ Forward

Physical Benefits
▸ Stretches the spine and shoulders
▸ Improves digestion
▸ Massages the abdominal organs and back
▸ Relieves lower back pain
▸ Opens the hips

Mental Benefit
▸ Relieves stress

Contraindications
▸ Knee injuries
▸ Hernia

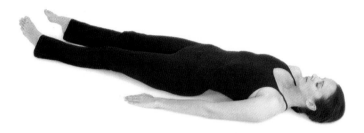

1 Lie on the floor with your legs extended.

Point your feet and keep your toes together.

Place your hands just below your knees.

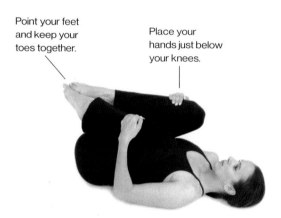

2 Bend your knees in toward your chest and separate your knees.

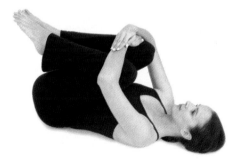

3 Draw your knees together and wrap your arms around your legs.

4 Roll to your right.

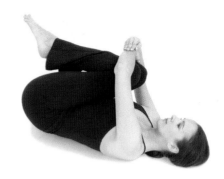

5 Roll to your left.

6 Repeat several times, then rest on your back or in Savasana (page 196).

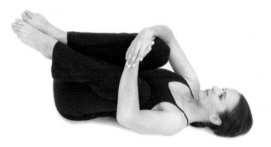

Reclining Hero

Supta Virasana

Counterpose
- Downward-Facing Dog (Adho Mukha Svanasana)

Drishti
- At ceiling
- Eyes closed

Physical Benefits
- Opens and releases the lower back
- Opens the chest for greater lung capacity
- Promotes the health and function of the hip, knee, and ankle joints
- Stimulates thyroid and parathyroid productivity
- Helps relieve menopausal discomfort
- Helps normalize high blood pressure
- Calms the nervous system

Mental Benefits
- Creates a feeling of grounding and stability
- Increases mental clarity
- Calms the mind

Contraindications
- Knee or ankle injury (use the gentle variation)
- Arthritis (use the gentle variation)
- Heart disease
- Pregnancy (after the first trimester use the gentle variation)

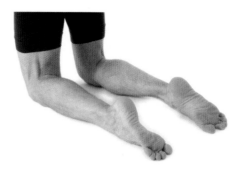

1 Standing on your knees, line up your feet and ankles straight back from your knees.

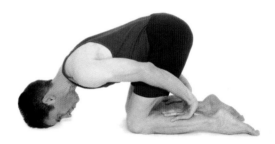

2 Smooth your calf muscles straight back with your hands, keeping even amounts of flesh on the insides and outsides of your legs. Rest your forehead on the floor if necessary.

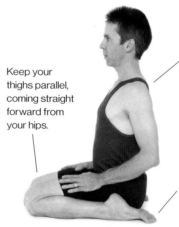

Keep your thighs parallel, coming straight forward from your hips.

Keep your shoulders back. Draw your shoulder blades down your back.

Rest the tops of your feet on the floor, keeping the ankle joints square. Press all ten toes into the floor to engage your foot and shin muscles.

3 Sit down between your ankles and extend from your low belly up through your head. Leave no space between your inner ankles and your hips.

4 Walk your hands behind you and slowly recline onto your forearms.

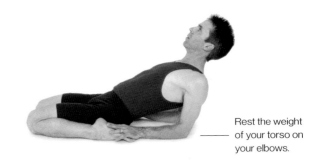

Rest the weight of your torso on your elbows.

5 Lower your torso all the way onto the floor and extend your arms up and over your head, keeping your shoulders down. Hold for as long as is comfortable. When you are ready, bring your arms down by your sides. Bend your elbows and slide them back to support your body weight. Draw your chin into your chest, press your elbows down, and bring your torso up. Stretch back into Downward-Facing Dog (see page 30).

Arch your pelvis slightly to create a curve in the low back. Then lengthen your tailbone and extend outward through your knees.

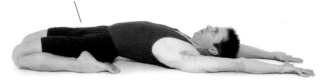

Gentle Variation

See Supported Hero (page 192). Follow steps 1 through 6 except if you are able to sit all the way to the floor, place a bolster or several folded blankets under your back. If you cannot sit to the floor, place the bolster under your hips and back.

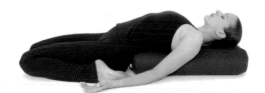

Other Variations

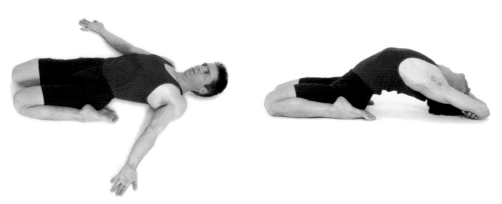

Reclining Big-Toe

Supta Padangusthasana

Counterpose

▶ Knees-to-Chest (Apanasana)

Drishti

▶ At ceiling

▶ At big toe

Physical Benefits

▶ Stimulates prostate gland

▶ Improves digestion

▶ Stretches hips, calves, and thighs

▶ Opens the hamstrings and psoas muscles

▶ Strengthens the knees

▶ Relieves menstrual and back discomfort

▶ Promotes reproductive health

▶ Strengthens arches of the feet

▶ Relieves sciatica and low back discomfort

Mental Benefits

▶ Calms the mind

▶ Relieves stress

Contraindications

▶ Headache

▶ High blood pressure (use the gentle variation)

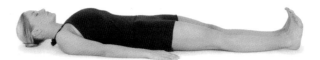

1 Lie flat on the floor; engage your legs and spread your toes. Anchor your upper thighs into the floor as firmly as possible. Arch your low back slightly to help get your thighs to descend.

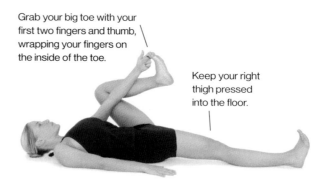

Grab your big toe with your first two fingers and thumb, wrapping your fingers on the inside of the toe.

Keep your right thigh pressed into the floor.

2 Bend your left knee and hold your big toe to the inside of your thigh.

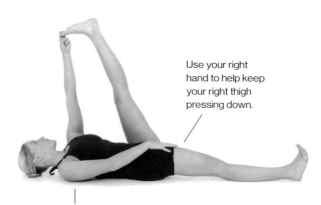

Use your right hand to help keep your right thigh pressing down.

Press your shoulders into the floor and slide your shoulder blades down your back toward your waist.

3 While holding on to your big toe, extend your left leg up, keeping your right thigh grounded into the floor. Extend from your pelvis through the sole of your left foot and press your left thigh away from your belly into your hamstrings.

Gentle Variation

Follow the instructions in steps 1 through 3, but use a strap over the sole of your foot. Hold the end of the strap with one hand.

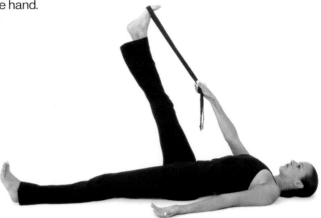

Reclining Bound-Angle

Supta Baddha Konasana

Counterposes

▷ Corpse (Savasana)
▷ Knees-to-Chest
  (Apanasana)

Drishti

▷ Eyes closed

Physical Benefits

▷ Improves digestion and
  circulation
▷ Keeps the prostate, kidneys,
  and urinary tract healthy
▷ Prevents varicose veins
▷ Promotes reproductive
  health
▷ Opens the chest
▷ Reduces fatigue and
  relieves headaches

Mental Benefits

▷ Helps draw the senses
  inward
▷ Relieves mild depression,
  stress, and anxiety

Contraindications

▷ Knee or groin injury (use the
  gentle variation)
▷ Low back pain (use the
  gentle variation)

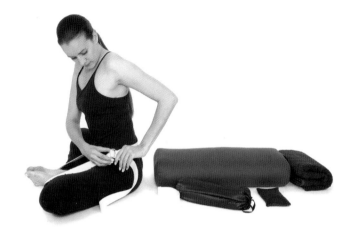

1 Sit at the edge of a large flat bolster. Bring the soles of your feet together and let your knees fall to the side. Drape a strap around your low back and over your thighs, around the front of your body and under your feet. Thread the strap and tighten until it is comfortably supported across your sacrum.

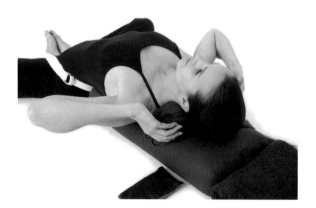

2 Slowly recline onto the bolster, adjusting the props as needed.

3 If desired, place a neck support or rolled towel under your neck and place an eye pillow across your closed eyes.

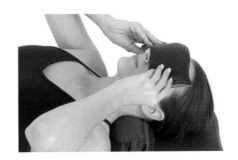

4 Relax into the pose and breathe slowly and evenly.

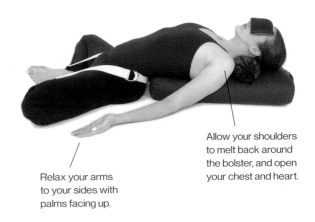

Allow your shoulders to melt back around the bolster, and open your chest and heart.

Relax your arms to your sides with palms facing up.

Gentle Variation

Follow steps 1 through 4, but place blankets or blocks under your knees or thighs to alleviate strain.

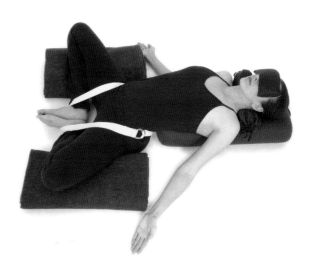

Reclining Open-Leg Spinal Twist

Jathara Parivartanasana

Counterpose
- Knees-to-Chest (Apanasana)

Drishti
- Eyes closed
- Beyond extended fingertips

Physical Benefits
- Stretches the spine and shoulders
- Improves digestion and circulation
- Massages the abdominal organs
- Strengthens low back
- Relieves lower backache, neck pain, and sciatica
- Opens hips

Mental Benefit
- Helps relieve stress, mild depression, and anxiety

Contraindications
- Low blood pressure
- Menstruation

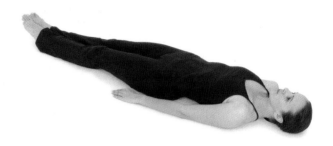

1 Lie on your back and extend your legs.

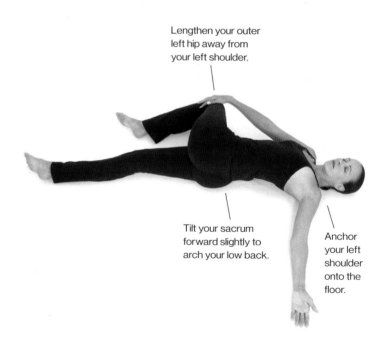

Lengthen your outer left hip away from your left shoulder.

Tilt your sacrum forward slightly to arch your low back.

Anchor your left shoulder onto the floor.

2 Draw your left leg up and twist it across your body, holding it with your right hand.

3 To deepen the twist, bend your right leg and reach for your foot with your left hand, drawing the heel in toward your hips.

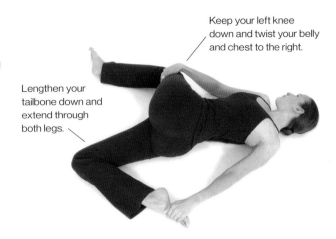

Keep your left knee down and twist your belly and chest to the right.

Lengthen your tailbone down and extend through both legs.

Gentle Variation

Keep your legs together on the same side of your body.

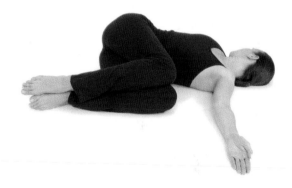

Other Variation

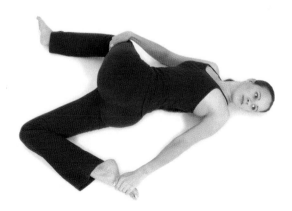

Supported Bridge

Salamba Setu Bandha Sarvangasana

Counterpose
▶ Knees-to-Chest
   (Apanasana)

Drishti
▶ At ceiling
▶ Eyes closed

Physical Benefits
▶ Alleviates low back
   discomfort
▶ Opens the heart, chest,
   neck, and spine
▶ Increases circulation in
   digestive and reproductive
   organs
▶ Stimulates pituitary, thyroid,
   and parathyroid gland
   function
▶ Helps alleviate sciatica
▶ Relieves menstrual
   discomfort
▶ Helps relieve asthma, high
   blood pressure, and sinusitis

Mental Benefits
▶ Stimulates the nervous
   system
▶ Reduces stress, mild
   depression, and anxiety

Contraindications
▶ Pregnancy (after the
   second trimester)
▶ Neck or spinal injury

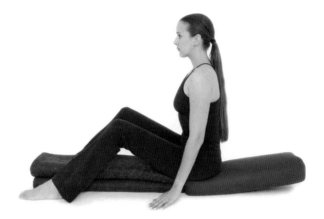

1 With a straight spine, sit near the middle of two bolsters or blankets that have been stacked end to end.

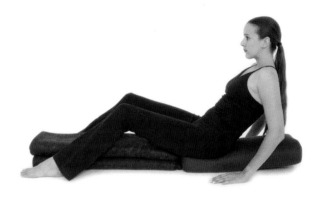

2 Using your hands as support, begin to slowly lower your body down on to the bolsters.

3 Place your hands flat along the side of the support and gently begin to recline. Keep your shoulders, neck, and head on the floor.

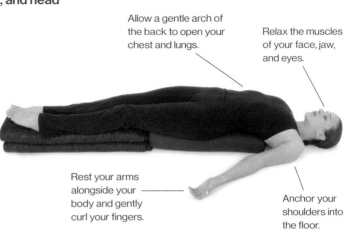

Allow a gentle arch of the back to open your chest and lungs.

Relax the muscles of your face, jaw, and eyes.

Rest your arms alongside your body and gently curl your fingers.

Anchor your shoulders into the floor.

Supported Hero

Supta Salamba Virasana

Counterpose

▶ Downward-Facing Dog
(Adho Mukha Svanasana)

Drishti

▶ Eyes closed

▶ Upward

Physical Benefits

▶ Opens and releases the lower back

▶ Promotes the health and function of the hip, knee, and ankle joints

▶ Stimulates thyroid and parathyroid productivity

▶ Helps relieve menopausal discomfort

▶ Therapeutic for high blood pressure

Mental Benefits

▶ Creates a feeling of grounding and stability

▶ Calms the mind

▶ Reduces stress, mild depression and anxiety

Contraindications

▶ Knee or ankle injury (use the gentle variation)

▶ Arthritis (use the gentle variation)

▶ Pregnancy (first trimester; use additional props)

▶ Heart disease

▶ Pregnancy (after the first trimester)

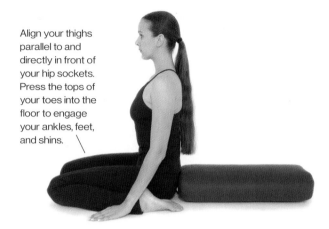

Align your thighs parallel to and directly in front of your hip sockets. Press the tops of your toes into the floor to engage your ankles, feet, and shins.

1 Bend your knees and sit on the floor with your heels at the outer edge of your hips. Place a large, flat bolster at the edge of your hips behind your body.

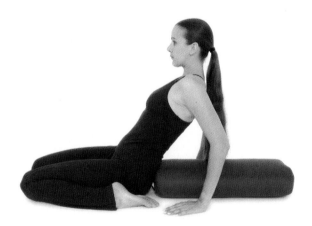

2 Bend your elbows and recline onto the bolster, keeping your spine lengthened.

3 Rest on the bolster with your arms by your sides. Allow your shoulders to melt back around the bolster.

4 Once supported, relax and melt into the pose, focusing on your breath.

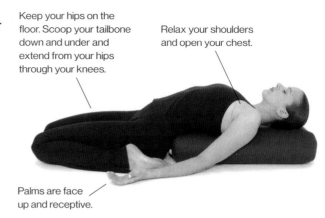

Keep your hips on the floor. Scoop your tailbone down and under and extend from your hips through your knees.

Relax your shoulders and open your chest.

Palms are face up and receptive.

Gentle Variation

Follow steps 1 through 3 except place the bolster under your hips and back.

Child's Pose

Balasana

Drishti

▶ Eyes closed

Physical Benefits

▶ Alleviates head, neck, and chest pain

▶ Opens the pelvic floor, hips, and low back

▶ Stretches ankles, knees, and hips

▶ Opens the upper back

Mental Benefits

▶ Calms the mind

▶ Reduces stress

▶ Lessens fatigue

Contraindications

▶ Pregnancy (keep the knees apart and do not place pressure on the abdominal region)

▶ Ankle, knee, or hip injury

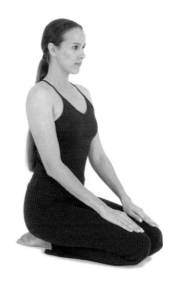

1 Sit on your heels with your shoulders above your hips.

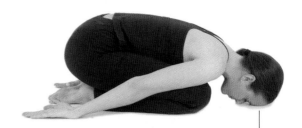

Rest your forehead on the floor, soften your face.

2 Bow forward and gently place your chest on your thighs.

3 As an option, bring your arms forward. Walk your fingertips forward and away from your shoulders.

Lengthen the sides of your body by extending from your hips to your shoulders.

Relax your arms to the floor.

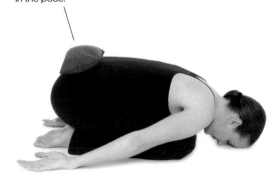

4 As an option, place a small sandbag or bolster on your low back. The pressure will relax your lower back muscles.

The prop should be heavy enough to feel, but light enough that it does not take away from your ability to relax and restore in the pose.

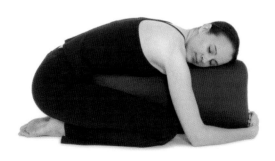

Gentle Variation

Follow the instructions in steps 1 through 4 but use a bolster to support your torso adjusting it as needed. Separate your knees to accommodate the bolster.

Corpse

Savasana

Drishti
▶ Eyes closed

Physical Benefits
▶ Lowers blood pressure
▶ Relaxes and rejuvenates the body
▶ Reduces fatigue

Mental Benefits
▶ Reduces stress, mild depression, and anxiety
▶ Reduces insomnia
▶ Calms and centers the mind

Contraindications
▶ Pregnancy (use the gentle variation or relax onto either side of the body with the knees drawn toward the chest)
▶ Low back or spinal injuries (use the gentle variation)

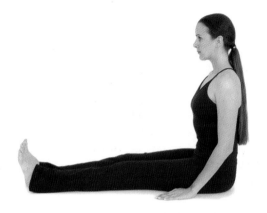

1 Sit with your legs extended and your hands by your sides.

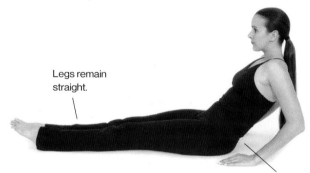

Legs remain straight.

As you lean back, keep your spine straight.

2 Support yourself with your arms as you recline onto the floor.

3 Lie flat on your back.

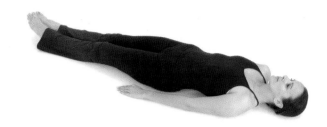

4 Relax your legs and allow your toes to roll out toward either side of the body. Move your arms 12 to 15 inches away from your sides with your hands on the floor and your palms face up. Soften completely into the floor.

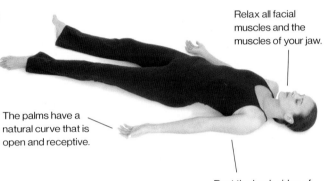

Relax all facial muscles and the muscles of your jaw.

The palms have a natural curve that is open and receptive.

Rest the back sides of your shoulders into the floor, opening your chest.

Gentle Variation

Follow steps 1 through 4, but place a bolster under your knees to support your low back.

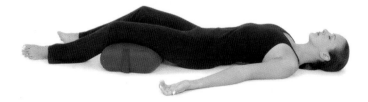

chapter 11

Hatha Yoga Routines

The yoga *asanas* described in this book are of great benefit when practiced individually. Once you become familiar with the poses it is advantageous to do them in a sequential series. This chapter introduces a series of asanas that collectively make up a routine similar to those you might experience in a yoga class. The routines provide a sequence or flow to your yoga practice that allows you to coordinate your breath with your movement. Along with conscious breath and movement you'll gain a greater sensitivity to your physical and energy body and the relationship between them. It is this awareness that is the essence of alignment.

The routines also help to bring the whole practice together by making a mindful connection between one pose and the next. Yoga is not only what happens during the pose but also what happens before and after the pose. Mindful movement from pose to pose will help you to center and make your yoga experience a moving meditation.

Please note that there are some poses in the routines that are not described in the text of this book. Therefore, it is recommended that you master similar poses from the book where possible to prepare yourself for these routines.

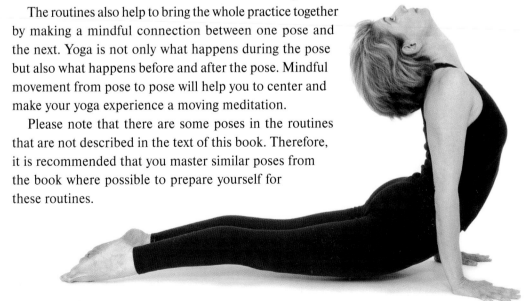

Gentle Yoga I

The postures in this routine provide maximum relaxation and can be performed by yoga students of all levels. Perform the routine in a quiet room with no distractions. Remain in each pose as long as it feels comfortable. Pay attention to your breath and notice the thoughts that will naturally flow in and out of your awareness like clouds floating in the sky. If you become distracted during your practice, return your attention to your breath. Conclude with Savasana (Corpse) for a minimum of 10 minutes. As you perform Gentle Yoga II on the next page, rest in Savasana, on your stomach, or in Child's Pose if necessary before proceeding to the next pose.

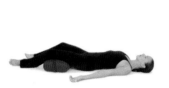

Supported Corpse
Supported Savasana
page 196

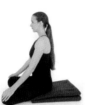

Sage
(variation)
Siddhasana
page 176

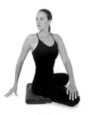

Gentle Spinal Twist
(variation)
page 122

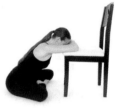

Supported Forward
Bend

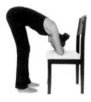

Standing Forward Bend
Uttanasana
page 138

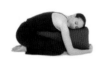

Supported Child's Pose
Balasana
page 194

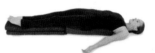

Supported Bridge
Salamba Setu Bandha
Sarvangasana
page 190

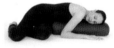

Supported Spinal Twist

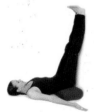

Legs-Up-the-Wall
Viparita Karani
page 94

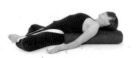

Reclining Bound-Angle
Supta Baddha Konasana
page 186

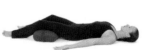

Supported Corpse
Supported Savasana
page 196

Gentle Yoga II

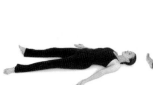

Corpse
Savasana
page 196

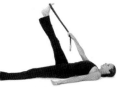

Reclining Big-Toe
Supta Padangusthasana
page 184

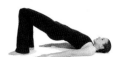

Bridge
Setu Banda
Sarvangasana
page 106

Knees-to-Chest
Apanasana
page 180

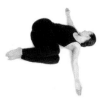

Reclining Spinal Twist
Jathara
Parivartanasana
page 124

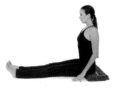

Staff Pose
Dandasana
page 170

Seated Forward Bend
Paschimottanasana
page 136

Lying on belly

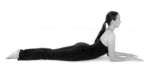

Cobra
(variation)
Bhujangasana
page 100

Child's Pose
Balasana
page 194

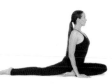

Pigeon
Eka Pada
Rajakapotasana
page 118

Staff Pose
Dandasana
page 170

Gentle Spinal Twist
(variation)
page 122

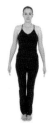

Mountain
Tadasana
page 28

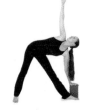

Extended Triangle
Utthita Trikonasana
page 34

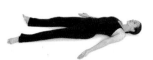

Corpse
Savasana
page 196

201

Yoga for Flexibility I

This routine includes postures to increase and maintain strength and flexibility. It starts with a standing series followed by hip openers, backbends, and a cool down. Coordinate the postures with your breath in the same manner as in the salutation series (see pages 210 to 216).

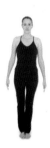

Mountain
Tadasana
page 28

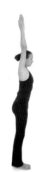

Mountain (arms up)
Tadasana
page 28

Standing Forward Bend
Uttanasana
page 138

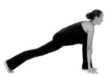

Lunge

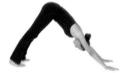

Downward-Facing Dog
Adho Mukha Svanasana
page 30

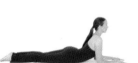

Cobra
(variation)
Bhujangasana
page 100

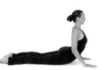

Cobra
Bhujangasana
page 100

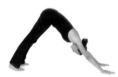

Downward-Facing Dog
Adho Mukha
Svanasana
page 30

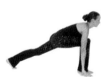

Lunge

Standing Forward Bend
Uttanasana
page 138

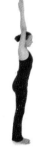

Mountain
(arms overhead)
Tadasana
page 28

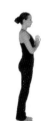

Mountain
(hands in Namaste)
Tadasana
page 28

Yoga for Flexibility I

(continued)

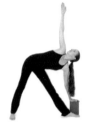

Extended Triangle
Utthita Trikonasana
page 34

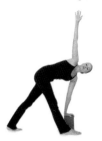

Revolved Triangle
Parivrtta Trikonasana
page 44

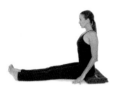

Staff Pose
Dandasana
page 170

Cow Face
Gomukhasana
page 168

Child's Pose
Balasana
page 194

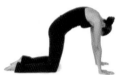

Cat
page 116

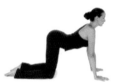

Cow
page 116

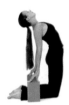

Camel
Ustrasana
page 104

Bridge
Setu Banda
Sarvangasana
page 106

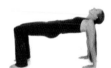

Intense front body
stretch, Inclined Plane
Purvottanasana
page 78

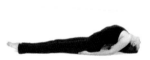

Fish
Matsyasana
page 114

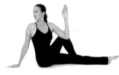

Seated Spinal Twist I
(variation)
Marichysana I
page 130

Staff Pose
Dandasana
page 170

Seated Forward Bend
Paschimottanasana
page 136

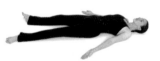

Corpse
Savasana
page 196

Yoga for Flexibility II

This routine includes postures to increase and maintain flexibility. It starts slowly building in intensity, peaks with challenging backbends, and ends with cooling postures. Coordinate the postures with your breath in the same manner as in the salutation series (see pages 210 to 216).

Child's Pose
Balasana
page 194

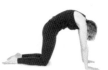

Exhale, Cat
page 116

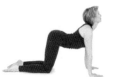

Inhale, Cow
page 116

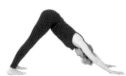

Exhale, Downward-
Facing Dog
Adho Mukha Svanasana
page 30

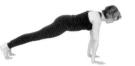

Inhale, Plank

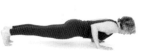

Exhale, Four-Limbed
Staff
Chaturanga Dandasana
page 86

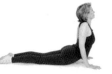

Exhale, Cobra, inhale
Bhujangasana
page 100

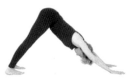

Exhale, Downward-
Facing Dog
Adho Mukha Svanasana
page 30

Inhale, Camel
Ustrasana
page 104

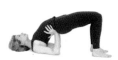

Inhale, Bridge, exhale
Setu Banda
Sarvangasana
page 106

Inhale, Upward-
Facing Bow
Urdva Dhanurasana,
exhale
page 112

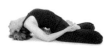

Inhale, Fish, exhale
Matsyasana
page 114

Exhale, cross-legged
Seated Spinal Twist I
(variation)
Marichyasana I
page 130

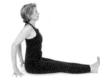

Inhale, Staff Pose
Dandasana
page 170

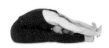

Exhale, Seated Forward
Bend, inhale
Paschimottanasana
page 136

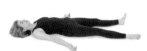

Exhale, Corpse
Savasana
page 196

Vinyasa Yoga I

Vinyasa Yoga I, II, and III are excellent routines for building strength and stamina. Concentrate on ujjayi breathing to center yourself and link the poses together. Perform the sequence first for the right side, then repeat for the left side.

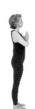

Mountain
(hands in Namaste)
Tadasana
page 28

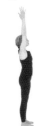

Inhale, Mountain
(arms overhead)
Tadasana
page 28

Exhale, Standing
Forward Bend
Uttanasana
page 138

Inhale, lengthen the spine

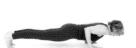

Exhale, Four-Limbed
Staff
Chaturanga Dandasana
page 86

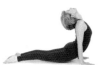

Inhale, Upward-
Facing Dog
Urdhva Mukha Svanasana
page 102

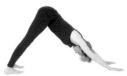

Exhale, Downward-
Facing Dog
Adho Mukha Svanasana
page 30

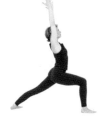

Inhale, Warrior I
Virabhadrasana I
page 40

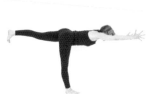

Exhale, Warrior III
Virabhadrasana III
page 70

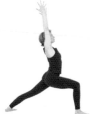

Inhale, Warrior I
Virabhadrasana I
page 40

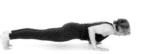

Exhale, Four-Limbed Staff
Chaturanga Dandasana
page 86

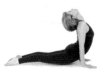

Inhale, Upward-Facing Dog
Urdhva Mukha Svanasana
page 102

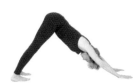

Exhale, Downward-
Facing Dog
Adho Mukha
Svanasana
page 30

Exhale, Standing
Forward Bend
Uttanasana
page 138

Inhale, Mountain
(arms overhead)
Tadasana
page 28

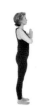

Exhale, Mountain
(hands in Namaste)
Tadasana
page 28

205

Vinyasa Yoga II

The Vinyasa Yoga II routine combines saluation flow with powerful standing poses to build strength and endurance. Concentrate on ujjayi breathing to link the poses together. Perform the sequence first for the right side, then repeat for the left side.

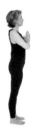

Mountain
(hands in Namaste)
Tadasana
page 28

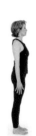

Exhale, Mountain
(arms at sides)
Tadasana
page 28

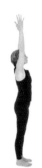

Inhale, Mountain
(arms overhead)
Tadasana
page 28

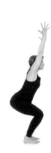

Exhale, Chair, inhale
Utkatasana
page 46

Exhale, Standing
Forward Bend
Uttanasana
page 138

Inhale, lengthen the spine

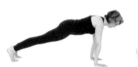

Exhale, Plank, inhale

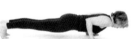

Exhale, Four-Limbed
Staff
Chaturanga Dandasana
page 86

Inhale, Upward-
Facing Dog
Urdhva Mukha
Svanasana
page 102

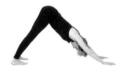

Exhale, Downward-
Facing Dog
Adho Mukha Svanasana
page 30

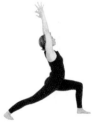

Inhale, Warrior I
Virabhadrasana I
page 40

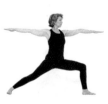

Exhale, Warrior II
Virabhadrasana II
page 36

206

Vinyasa Yoga II

(continued)

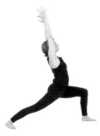

Inhale, Warrior I
Virabhadrasana I
page 40

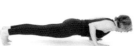

Exhale, Plank, inhale

Exhale, Four-Limbed
Staff
Chaturanga Dandasana
page 86

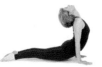

Inhale, Upward-
Facing Dog
Urdhva Mukha Svanasana
page 102

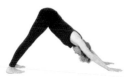

Exhale, Downward-
Facing Dog
Adho Mukha Svanasana
page 30

Inhale, step the feet to
the hands and lengthen
the spine

Exhale, Standing
Forward Bend
Uttanasana
page 138

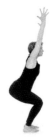

Inhale, Chair, exhale
Utkatasana
page 46

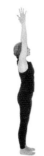

Inhale, Mountain
(arms overhead)
Tadasana
page 28

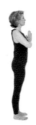

Exhale, Mountain
(hands in Namaste)
Tadasana
page 28

Vinyasa Yoga III

Vinyasa Yoga III is an excellent routine designed to build strength and stamina with a focus on twists. Concentrate on ujjayi breathing to link the poses together. Perform the sequence first for the right side, then repeat for the left side.

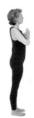

Inhale, Mountain
(hands in Namaste)
Tadasana
page 28

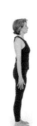

Exhale, Mountain
(arms at sides)
Tadasana
page 28

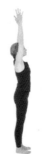

Inhale, Moutain
(arms overhead)
Tadasana
page 28

Exhale, Standing
Forward Bend
Uttanasana
page 138

Inhale, lengthen the spine

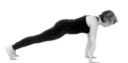

Exhale, Plank, inhale

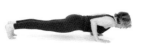

Exhale, Four-Limbed
Staff
Chaturanga Dandasana
page 86

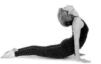

Inhale, Upward-
Facing Dog
Urdhva Mukha
Svanasana
page 102

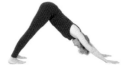

Exhale, Downward-
Facing Dog
Adho Mukha Svanasana
page 30

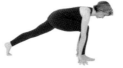

Inhale, Lunge

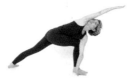

Inhale, Revolved Intense
Side-Stretch
Parivrtta
Parsvakonasana
page 54

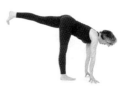

Inhale, place the hands
on the ground, lift the
opposite leg up

Vinyasa Yoga III

(continued)

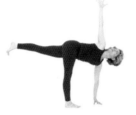

Exhale, inhale, Revolved Half Moon Parivrtta Ardha Chandrasana page 66

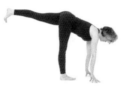

Exhale, bring both hands down under the shoulders

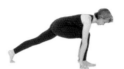

Inhale, exhale, Lunge

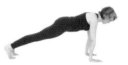

Inhale, Plank

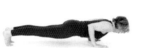

Exhale, Four-Limbed Staff Chaturanga Dandasana page 86

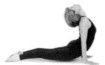

Inhale, Upward-Facing Dog Urdhva Mukha Svanasana page 102

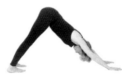

Exhale, Downward-Facing Dog Adho Mukha Svanasana page 30

Inhale, step the feet to the hands and lengthen the spine

Exhale, Standing Forward Bend Uttanasana page 138

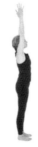

Inhale, Mountain (arms overhead) Tadasana page 28

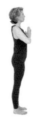

Exhale, Mountain (hands in Namaste) Tadasana page 28

Sun Salutation I

Sun Salutation I is an excellent warm-up routine for most yoga practices or to start your day. It is also an excellent stand alone routine that can be completed in about a minute. Concentrate on the breathing throughout the routine. Once you have completed the series with one leg, repeat using the other leg.

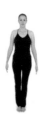

Mountain
Tadasana
page 28

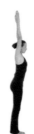

Inhale, Mountain
(arms overhead)
Tadasana
page 28

Exhale, Standing
Forward Bend
Uttanasana
page 138

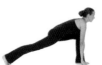

Exhale, Lunge

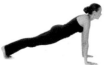

Inhale, Plank

Inhale, exhale, Cobra
Bhujangasana
page 100

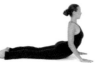

Exhale, Cobra
Bhujangasana
page 100

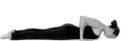

Inhale, exhale, Cobra
Bhujangasana
page 100

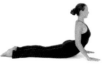

Inhale, Cobra
Bhujangasana
page 100

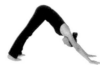

Exhale, Downward-
Facing Dog
Adho Mukha Svanasana
page 30

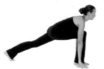

Inhale, Lunge

Exhale, Standing
Forward Bend
Uttanasana
page 138

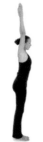

Inhale, Mountain
(arms overhead)
Tadasana
page 28

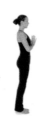

Exhale, Mountain
(hands in Namaste)
Tadasana
page 28

Sun Salutation II

Sun Salutation II is also an excellent warm-up routine for most yoga practices and can serve as a stand alone routine for building stamina, strength, and flexibility. It can be completed in about a minute. Concentrate on ujjayi breathing to link the poses together.

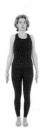
Exhale, Mountain
Tadasana
page 28

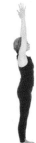
Inhale, Mountain
(arms overhead)
Tadasana
page 28

Exhale, Standing
Forward Bend
Uttanasana
page 138

Inhale, lengthen the spine

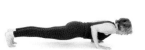
Exhale, Four-Limbed
Staff
Chaturanga Dandasana
page 86

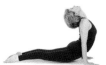
Inhale, Upward-
Facing Dog
Urdhva Mukha
Svanasana
page 102

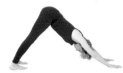
Exhale, Downward-
Facing Dog
Adho Mukha Svanasana
page 30

Inhale, lengthen the spine

Exhale, Standing
Forward Bend
Uttanasana
page 138

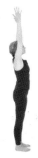
Inhale, Mountain
(arms overhead)
Tadasana
page 28

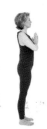
Exhale, Mountain
(hands in Namaste)
Tadasana
page 28

Moon Salutation I

This is primarily a back-bending salutation. Coordinate your movements with your breath. If you need to rest, remain in Child's Pose for 10 breaths before continuing with the series. This series is shown leading with the right side. Complete the entire series and then repeat leading with your left side.

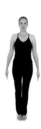

Exhale, Mountain
Tadasana
page 28

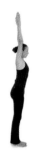

Inhale, Mountain
(arms overhead)
Tadasana
page 28

Exhale, Standing
Forward Bend
Uttanasana
page 138

Inhale, Garland
(variation)
Malasana
page 150

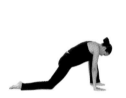

Exhale, place your hands
down, Lunge

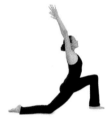

Inhale, Crescent Lunge,
(variation)
Alanasana
page 38

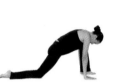

Exhale, Lunge

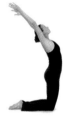

Inhale, Camel (variation)
Ustrasana
page 104

Exhale, Child's Pose
Balasana
page 194

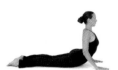

Inhale, forward Cobra
Bhujangasana
page 100

Exhale, Child's Pose
Balasana
page 194

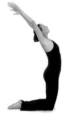

Inhale, Camel
(variation), exhale
Ustrasana
page 104

Moon Salutation I

(continued)

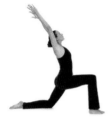

Inhale, Crescent Lunge,
(variation)
Alanasana
page 38

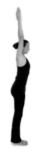

Exhale, Lunge

Inhale, Garland
(variation)
Malasana
page 150

Exhale, Standing
Forward Bend
Uttanasana
page 138

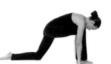

Inhale, Mountain
(arms overhead)
Tadasana
page 28

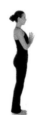

Exhale, Mountain
(hands in Namaste)
Tadasana
page 28

Moon Salutation II

This is a full range series incorporating forward-, side-, and back-bending poses. Coordinate your movements with ujjayi breathing. If you need to rest, remain in Child's Pose for 10 breaths before continuing with the series.

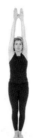

Exhale, Mountain
Tadasana
page 28

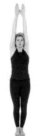

Inhale, Mountain
(thumbs linked together,
arms overhead)
Tadasana
page 28

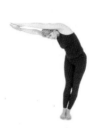

Exhale, bow to the side
and slightly forward

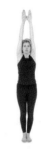

Inhale, Mountain
(thumbs linked together,
arms overhead)
Tadasana
page 28

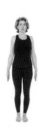

Exhale, bow to the other
side and slightly forward.

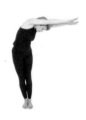

Inhale, Mountain
(thumbs linked together,
arms overhead)
Tadasana
page 28

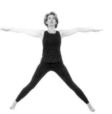

Exhale, step wide
with arms at the side,
and inhale.

Exhale, Standing
Intense Spread-Leg
Pose
Prasarita
Padottanasana
page 48

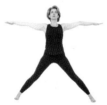

Inhale, lift the torso

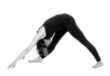

Exhale, Intense Side
Stretch
Parsvottanasana
page 54

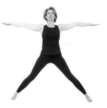

Inhale, lift the torso

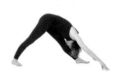

Exhale, Intense Side Stretch
Parsvottanasana
page 54

Moon Salutation II

(continued)

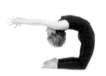

Inhale, lift the torso, exhale

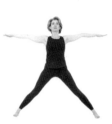

Inhale, Mountain (arms overhead) Tadasana page 28

Exhale, Standing Forward Bend, inhale Uttanasana page 138

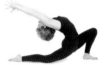

Exhale, step back, inhale, arms up

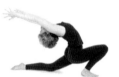

Exhale, bring the left leg, kneel, inhale, reach up, and arch the back, Camel (variation) Ustrasana page 104

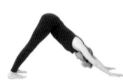

Exhale, step the right foot forward, inhale, arms up

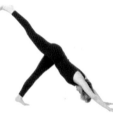

Exhale, Downward-Facing Dog Adho Mukha Svanasana page 30

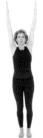

Inhale, lift your right leg up in line with your spine Downward-Facing Dog (variation) Adho Mukha Svanasana page 30

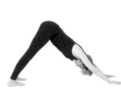

Exhale, Downward-Facing Dog Adho Mukha Svanasana page 30

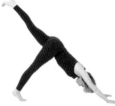

Inhale, lift your left leg up in line with your spine Downward-Facing Dog (variation) Adho Mukha Svanasana page 30

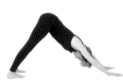

Exhale, Downward-Facing Dog Adho Mukha Svanasana page 30

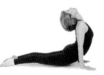

Inhale, Upward-Facing Dog Urdhva Mukha Svanasana page 102

Moon Salutation II

(continued)

Exhale, Child's Pose
Balasana
page 194

Inhale, Garland
(variation), exhale
Malasana
page 150

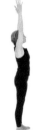

Inhale, Mountain
(arms overhead)
Tadasana
page 28

Exhale, Standing
Forward Bend
Uttanasana
page 138

Inhale, lengthen the spine

Exhale, Standing
Forward Bend
Uttanasana
page 138

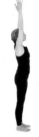

Inhale, Mountain
(arms overhead)
Tadasana
page 28

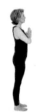

Exhale, Mountain
(hands in Namaste)
Tadasana
page 28

Suggested Readings

Baptiste, Baron. 2002. *Journey Into Power*. New York: Fireside.

Bouanchaud, Bernard. 1997. *The Essence of Yoga*. Portland: Rudra Press.

Browning-Miller, Elise, and Carol Blackman. 1999. *Life Is a Stretch*. St. Paul: Llewellyn.

Desikachar, T.K.V. 1995. *The Heart of Yoga*. Rochester, NY: Inner Traditions International.

Durgananda, Swami. 2001. *The Heart of Meditation*. South Fallsburg, NY: Siddha Yoga.

Frawley, David. 1999. *Yoga & Ayurveda*. Twin Lakes, WI: Lotus Press.

Friend, John. 1999. *Anusara Yoga Teacher Training Manual*. Spring, TX: Anusara Press.

Hirschi, Gertrude. 2000. *Mudras: Yoga in Your Hands*. Boston, MA: Red Wheel/Weiser.

Iyengar, B.K.S. 1977. *Light on Yoga: Yoga Dipika*. New York: Schoken Books.

Iyengar, B.K.S. 1992. *Light on Pranayama: The Yogic Art of Breathing*. New York: Crossroads.

Judith, Anodea. 2002. *Wheels of Life: A Users Guide to the Chakra System*. St. Paul: Llewellyn.

Khalsa, Dharma Singh, and Cameron Stauth. 2001. *Meditation as Medicine*. New York: Simon & Schuster.

Lad, Dr. Vasant. 1984. *Ayurveda—The Science of Self-Healing*. Twin Lakes, WI: Lotus Press.

Lasater, Judith. 1995. *Relax and Renew*. Berkeley: Rodmell Press.

LeShan, Lawrence. 1974. *How to Meditate*. New York: Little, Brown & Company.

Mehta, Silva, et al. 1990. *Yoga: The Iyengar Way*. New York: Knopf.

Olivelle, Patrick. 1996. *Upanishads*. New York: Oxford University Press.

Schifman, Erich. 1996. *Yoga: The Spirit and Practice of Moving Into Stillness*. New York: Pocket.

Resources

Yoga Schools—
North American Headquarters

Ananda Yoga
J. Donald Walters (Kriyananda), founder
14618 Tyler Foote Rd.
Nevada City, CA 95959
(800) 346-5350
www.expandinglight.org

Anusara Yoga
John Friend, founder
9400 Grogans Mill Rd., Ste. 200
The Woodlands, TX 77380
(888) 398-9642
www.anusara.com

Ashtanga Yoga
Sri Pattabi Jois, founder
David Swenson, Ashtanga Yoga Productions
P.O. Box 5099
Austin, TX 78763
In USA: (800) 684-6927
In Canada: (604) 732-6111
www.ashtanga.net

Babaji's Kriya Hatha Yoga
Marshall Govindan, founder
196 Mountain Rd., P.O. Box 90
Eastman, Quebec, Canada J0E 1P0
(888) 252-YOGA
www.babaji.ca

Baptiste Power Yoga Institute
Baron Baptiste, founder
P.O. Box 400279
Cambridge, MA 02140
(617) 441-2144
www.baronbaptiste.com

Bikram Yoga
Bikram Choudhury, founder
1862 S. La Cienega Blvd.
Los Angeles, CA 90035
(310) 854-5800
www.bikramyoga.com

Himalayan Institute
Swami Rama, founder
RR1 Box 1127
Honesdale, PA 18431-9706
(800) 822-4547
www.himalayaninstitute.org

Integral Yoga Institute
Sri Swami Satchidananda, founder
Route 1, Box 1720
Buckingham, VA 23921
(434) 969-3121
www.yogaville.org

Iyengar Yoga Institute of San Francisco
B.K.S. Iyengar, founder
2404 27th Ave.
San Francisco, CA 94116
(415) 753-0909
www.iyisf.org

International Sivananda Yoga Vedanta Centers
Swami Vishnu-devananda, founder
5178, St-Laurent Blvd.
Montreal, Canada H2T 1R8
Quebec, Canada
In USA: (800) 783-YOGA
In Canada: (800) 263-YOGA
www.sivananda.org

Kripalu Center
Yogi Amrit Desai, founder
P.O. Box 793
Lenox, MA 01240
(800) 741-7353
www.kripalu.org

3HO Kundalini Yoga Centers
Yogi Bhajan, founder
01A Ram Das Guru Place
Espanola, NM 87532
www.yogibhajan.com

Mount Madonna Center
Baba Hari Dass, founder
445 Summit Rd.
Watsonville, CA 95076
(408) 847-0406
www.mountmadonna.org

Tri Yoga
Kali Ray, founder
P.O. Box 6367
Malibu, CA 90264
(310) 589–0600
www.kaliraytriyoga.com

White Lotus Yoga
Ganga White, founder
2500 San Marcos Pass
Santa Barbara, CA 93105
(805) 964-1944
www.whitelotus.org

Sources for Yoga Props and Clothing

Most of the yoga supplies used for this book were obtained from Hugger Mugger Yoga Products.

Hugger Mugger Yoga Products
3937 South 500 West
Salt Lake City, UT 84123
 (800) 473-4888
www.huggermugger.com

Other sources for yoga supplies:

Asana
2118 Wilshire Blvd., Suite 850
Santa Monica, CA 90403
(888) 511-1144
asana2@earthlink.net

Bheka yoga supplies
(800) 366-4541
www.bheka.com

Blue Lotus Yoga Essentials
3120 Central Ave. SE
Albuquerque, NM 87106
(888) 645-4452
www.bluelotusyoga.com

The Sitting Room
(zafus and meditation supplies)
P.O. Box 885044
San Francisco, CA 94188
(800) 720-9642
www.yogamats.com

Tools for Yoga
P.O. Box 99
Chatham, NJ 07928
(973) 966-5311
www.yogapropshop.com

Yoga Pro
P.O. Box 7612
Ann Arbor, MI 48107
(800) 488-8414
www.yogapro.com

YogaSuperStore.com
6947 California St.
San Francisco, CA 94121
(866) 300-5298
www.yogasuperstore.com

Yoga Zone
3342 Melrose Ave. NW
Roanoke, VA 24017
(800) 264-9642
www.yogazone.com

Index of Asanas

Photographic Index by English Name

Alphabetical by Sanskrit Name

About the Authors

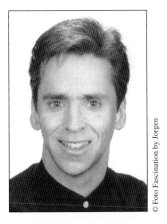

© Foto Fascination by Jorgen

Martin Kirk is a senior Anusara Yoga certified yoga instructor and a registered yoga teacher with Yoga Alliance. He has trained extensively with John Friend, Anusara Yoga founder, since 1994 and continues to apprentice with him nationally. Kirk and his wife, Jordan, are the founders of Yoga Village in Scottsdale, Arizona, and directors of teacher training. They lead workshops and yoga retreats worldwide.

With a master's degree in biomedical engineering, Kirk has a gift for teaching anatomy and therapeutics. He is frequently a special guest instructor at yoga teacher trainings. Kirk is a member of the Arizona Yoga Association.

Kirk lives in Scottsdale, Arizona, with his wife. He can be contacted via the Web at www.martinkirk.com or by e-mail at martin@yogavillage.net.

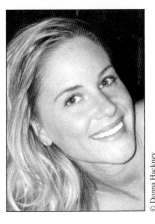

© Donna Hackney

Brooke Boon, RYT, is the founder and program director of Holy Yoga. She is an energetic and dedicated lover of yoga, healing, and the Lord. She creatively weaves spirituality, physical alignment, practical wisdom, and the Word into the fabric of her teaching. She has been blessed with the opportunity to be a leader in the Christian Yoga Movement while developing, branding, and implementing Holy Yoga classes across the country. Brooke has created and begun facilitating the Holy Yoga teacher training program which trains devoted teachers to inspire students to connect individually with Christ.

Brooke has a deep appreciation for the practice of yoga and connection to Christ as a collective and authentic path to wellness. "The love of the Lord and His Word has given this practice its power, flow, and grace. It is like nothing I have ever taught or been taught. It is a true form of worship."

Brooke lives in Phoenix, Arizona with her husband, Jarrett, and three children, Jory, Jace, and Brynn. You can connect with Brooke at www.holyyoga.net or by calling 866-737-HOLY.

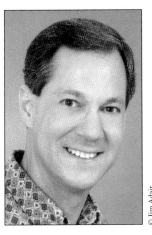

© Jim Adair

Daniel DiTuro was born in Phoenix, Arizona, and is a graduate of Arizona State University with a bachelor's degree in mechanical engineering. He has worked as a mechanical engineer since 1980. He developed an interest in the arts and photography at an early age and in 1986 started DiTuro Photography (www.diturophotography.com), specializing in commercial and portrait photography.

Following a shoulder injury in 1999, Daniel began practicing hatha yoga. Having discovered the therapeutic benefits and the misconceptions about this East Indian philosophy, he began working on a series of yoga and meditation photographs that evolved into the Yoga Project (www.diturophotography.com/typ).

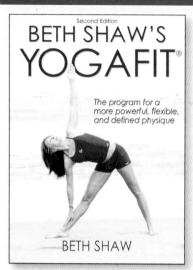
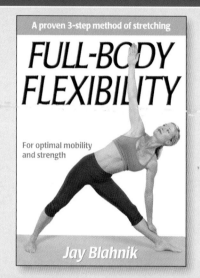